Walter Bockting, PhD
Sheila Kirk, MD
Editors

Transgender and HIV
Risks, Prevention, and Care

Pre-publication
REVIEW

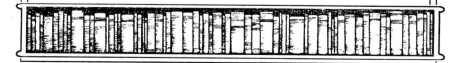

Transgender and HIV
Risks, Prevention, and Care

THE HAWORTH PRESS
Human Sexuality
Eli Coleman, PhD
Senior Editor

Transgender and HIV
Risks, Prevention, and Care

Walter Bockting, PhD
Sheila Kirk, MD
Editors

The Haworth Press®
New York • London • Oxford

The Haworth Press, Inc., 10 Alice Street, Binghamton, NY 13904–1580

All chapters, with the exception of Chapter 2, were previously published online in a special issue of the *International Journal of Transgenderism*, 3(1/2), 1999, <www.symposion.com/ijt>. Reprinted with permission of Symposion Publishing.

Cover design by Jennifer M. Gaska.

Cover photos © Debra Davis at the Program in Human Sexuality's Transgender HIV Prevention Workshop, funded by the American Foundation for AIDS Research, Grant No. 100108-12-EG. Reprinted with permission.

Library of Congress Cataloging-in-Publication Data

Transgender and HIV : risks, prevention, and care / Walter Bockting, Sheila Kirk, editors.
    p. cm.
    Includes bibliographical references and index.
    ISBN 0-7890-1267-7 (hard) — ISBN 0-7890-1268-5 (soft)
    1. AIDS (Disease) 2. Transsexuals—Diseases. I. Bockting, Walter O. II. Kirk, Sheila, M.D.
RA644.A25 T736 2001
616.97'92'00866—dc21

                                           00-063367

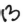

This book is dedicated to the memory
of Louis Graydon Sullivan,
one man who made a difference.

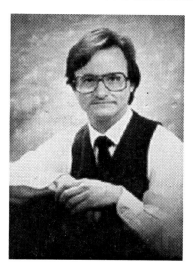

Lou Sullivan was born in a female body June 15, 1951, in Milwaukee, Wisconsin. From an early age, he struggled with the clash between his female body and his sense of himself as a gay man. In the early 1970s, he produced a newsletter for the Milwaukee gay scene and wrote for a number of gay and feminist publications. He moved to San Francisco with his boyfriend in the mid-1970s. He began his hormonal transition to a male body in 1978, and his relationship ended when he decided to seek chest reconstruction, which he had in 1980. Motivated by his awareness of the difficulty of finding reliable information about FTM transition, he produced his first informational booklet on FTMs for the Janus Information Facility, where he served as a volunteer.

Because of his sexual orientation as a gay man, he was refused genital reconstruction three times. Eventually he was able to find a surgeon who would work with him, and he had his genitals rendered to a masculine configuration in April 1986. He suffered many complications from that surgery, and he never really recovered. He was diagnosed with HIV in late 1986. Prejudice against the disease cost him his job, and he decided to devote the remainder of his life to developing social support for FTM transsexuals and cross-dressers, and to educating health care professionals about the process and dynamics of female-to-male transition. In the spring of 1987, he began a small FTM peer support group in San Francisco, and he also began publishing *The FTM Newsletter* in September of that same year. After a ragged start, meetings and newsletter issues became quarterly events.

Lou set the stage for the later development of the educational organization FTM International, and for the development of an international FTM community that does not condone judging people by their sexual orientation. Interested in history, he was a founding member of the Gay and Lesbian Historical Society of Northern California. He was a prolific letter writer who took the time to pay attention to each and every person he made contact with who sought information about cross-dressing, passing, or sex reassignment surgery. He was concerned that transsexual people remain aware that not everyone reaches the same life decisions in the same way or at the same moment, nor do the same issues or concerns motivate them all. He was instrumental in raising the level of discussion within professional circles concerning the separation of sexual orientation and gender identity, as well as the existence of FTM cross-dressers and gay-identified FTMs. He wrote two books: *Information for the FTM Cross Dresser and Transsexual* and *From Female to Male: The Life of Jack Bee Garland.*

Lou died March 2, 1991, at the age of thirty-nine. He was not widely known. The phenomenal growth of transgender awareness and the synergy between the GLB and T communities had not been fully explored. No conscious effort had yet been made to serve transgendered or transsexual people with AIDS. Lou Sullivan left behind a mailing list of about 230 names, a roll of stamps, the model of inclusion in his support group, and the ethic of service to a community he hoped would someday exist. Now it almost does. In life and since his death, he has been an inspiration for many transgender men, both gay and straight.

This volume is a fitting tribute to his efforts. He would be honored.

Jamison Green
Past President, FTM International, Inc.
San Francisco

CONTENTS

ABOUT THE EDITORS

Walter O. Bockting, PhD, is a licensed psychologist, Assistant Professor, and Coordinator of Transgender Services at the Program in Human Sexuality at the University of Minnesota in Minneapolis. He is also on the graduate faculty of the Center for Advanced Feminist Studies. His interests include transgender and transsexual identity, HIV/STD prevention, and the promotion of sexual health. He has presented at many national and international scientific conferences on sex, gender, and human sexuality.

Dr. Bockting is the author of *Transgender HIV Prevention: A Minnesota Response to a Global Health Concern* and the editor of *Gender Dysphoria: Interdisciplinary Approaches in Clinical Management* (Haworth) and the *International Journal of Transgenderism.* He is a member of the Board of Directors of the Harry Benjamin International Gender Dysphoria Association and the Society for the Scientific Study of Sexuality.

Sheila Kirk, MD, is the first transsexual surgeon to develop and direct a facility specializing in complete transgender surgical and medical care as well as the only transsexual physician worldwide who has performed genital reassignment surgeries. This unique position enables her to help those in the transgender community improve their overall physical and emotional well-being while providing insight and instruction to the medical professionals who administer their care.

Dr. Kirk is the author of *Feminizing Hormonal Therapy for the Transgendered; Masculinizing Hormonal Therapy for the Transgendered; Medical, Legal and Workplace Issues for the Transsexual;* and the *Physician's Guide to Transgendered Medicine.*

A leading authority on transgender issues, Dr. Kirk lectures extensively at universities, medical conferences, and symposiums, both nationally and internationally.

CONTRIBUTORS

Kristen Clements-Nolle, MPH, Epidemiologist, San Francisco Department of Public Health AIDS Office, San Francisco, California.

Eli Coleman, PhD, President, Harry Benjamin International Gender Dysphoria Association; Director, Program in Human Sexuality and Behavioral Science; Professor, Department of Family Practice and Community Health, University of Minnesota Medical School, Minneapolis, Minnesota.

Margaret Connors, PhD, Consultant, Boston, Massachusetts.

Rebecca Durkee, Transgender Education Specialist, Boston, Massachusetts.

Jamison Green, MFA, Past President, FTM International, Inc.; Chairman, Board of Directors, Gender Education and Advocacy, Inc., Oakland, California.

Douglas Hein, BA, Manager of Counseling, Testing, and Support Service, AIDS Program, Boston Public Health Commission, Boston, Massachusetts.

James A. Inciardi, PhD, Director, Center for Drug and Alcohol Studies, University of Delaware, New York City; Professor, Department of Sociology and Criminal Justice, University of Delaware; Adjunct Professor, Department of Epidemiology and Public Health, University of Miami School of Medicine, Miami, Florida; Guest Professor, Department of Psychiatry at the Federal University of Rio Grande do Sul, Porto Allegre, Brazil.

Nina Kammerer, PhD, **MPH,** Senior Researcher, Health and Addictions Research, Inc., Boston, Massachusetts; Affiliated Scholar, Women's Studies Program and Research Associate, Department of Anthropology, Brandeis University, Waltham, Massachusetts.

Michael Kirk, BFA, Founder of Enterprise, the FTM Center at Boston Medical Center, and the Lionheart Group, Boston, Massachusetts.

Kerrily Kitano, PhD, Consultant, San Francisco, California.

Emilia L. Lombardi, PhD, Research Sociologist, UCLA Drug Abuse Research Center, Los Angeles, California.

Rani Marx, PhD, MPH, Director, Epidemiology & Evaluation Section, San Francisco Department of Public Health AIDS Office, San Francisco, California.

Theresa Mason, PhD, Social Anthropologist, Abt Associates, Cambridge, Massachusetts.

Viviane K. Namaste, PhD, Coordinator, community-based transsexual health care project, CACTUS, Montréal, Canada.

Binh H. Pok, BA, PhD candidate, Graduate Center of the City University of New York, New York City.

Cathy J. Reback, PhD, Director of Prevention, Van Ness Recovery House, Friends Research Institute, Los Angeles, California.

B. R. Simon Rosser, PhD, MPH, Director, Community Health Professor, Program in Human Sexuality, Department of Family Practice and Community Health, University of Minnesota Medical School, Minneapolis, Minnesota; Visiting Behavioral Scientist, Division of HIV/AIDS Prevention—Intervention Research and Support, National Center for HIV, STD, and TB Prevention, Centers for Disease Control and Prevention, Atlanta, Georgia.

Hilary L. Surratt, MA, Associate Scientist, Center for Drug and Alcohol Studies, University of Delaware, New York City.

Paulo R. Telles, MD, PhD, Senior Researcher, Núcleo de Estudos e Pesquisas em Atenção ao Uso de Drogas, State University of Rio de Janeiro, Rio de Janeiro, Brazil.

Barbara E. Warren, PsyD, Director, Mental Health and Social Services, Lesbian and Gay Community Services Center, New York City.

Willy Wilkinson, MPH, Consultant, San Francisco, California.

A. Neal Wilson, MB, BS, FRCS (ED), FRCS (ENG), DO, RCOG, Clinical Assistant Professor of Surgery, Division of Plastic Surgery, Wayne State University School of Medicine; Vice Chief of Surgery and Chief of Plastic Surgery, Hutzel Hospital, Detroit Medical Center, Detroit, Michigan.

Foreword

Walter Bockting and Sheila Kirk are to be commended for compiling this outstanding collection of material on HIV/AIDS as it relates to the transgender community. Not only has there been a paucity of information regarding the revolutionary changes that have occurred within the transgender community, but very little literature has been published regarding HIV/AIDS and its impact on transgender individuals. This book clearly fills that void.

As many of the authors point out, stigma and discrimination places this population at severe risk for a number of health-related problems. Furthermore, failure to acknowledge these problems makes this health crisis even more catastrophic. Yet, out of this horror, the transgender community has demanded that its voice be heard and has emerged stronger. As a result, researchers have been able to alert health departments and funding agencies of the necessity to better understand the health care needs of this community and to provide access to such care. These efforts are reflected in this collection.

It is only fitting that this volume be dedicated to Lou Sullivan, a transgender activist who died of AIDS. He helped galvanize the FTM transgender community and was also outspoken about his HIV status. His voice echoes throughout these pages.

This book is bound to enlighten anyone about the transgender community. Although the focus is on HIV prevention, the authors note that HIV-prevention programming must address the wider context of these individuals' lives. Thus, this book lends itself to more than HIV prevention programming and is a start toward creating better health care in general (from prevention to tertiary care). It is also a testimony to collaboration as an essential means to providing better health care. However, this will not be accomplished until further changes occur to eliminate social stigma and discrimination. We need societal changes as a primary prevention strategy to reduce the risk of HIV infection and other health risks.

I hope that everyone who reads this book will take up the challenge. Change can start with one voice such as Lou Sullivan's, but it will take many more to make a chorus. We must work in collaboration and harmony.

Eli Coleman, PhD
President, Harry Benjamin
International Gender Dysphoria Association;
Professor and Director,
Program in Human Sexuality,
Department of Family Practice
and Community Health,
University of Minnesota Medical School

Preface

Until recently, the impact of the HIV/AIDS epidemic on the transgender community was largely ignored. Despite reports of high prevalence of HIV among certain subgroups of the transgender population, targeted prevention was virtually nonexistent (Bockting, Robinson, and Rosser, 1998). This began to change when, in 1992, the University of Minnesota Program in Human Sexuality received a grant from the American Foundation for AIDS Research to develop one of the first transgender-specific HIV prevention programs. Since then, the program has received requests for materials from communities around the world. From these interactions emerged a network of researchers, service providers, and community leaders engaged in transgender-specific HIV prevention efforts. We invited representatives of these efforts to disseminate their findings and to share their expertise by contributing to this volume.

The growing awareness of the need for HIV prevention to target transgenders has already begun to bear fruit. In 1994, as part of Minnesota's statewide HIV community planning process, members of the local transgender community participated in focus groups that identified several HIV risk factors: invisibility, poverty, shame, low self-esteem, loneliness, and sharing needles for hormone or silicone injection (Minnesota Department of Health, 1994). We learned that many transgenders view acceptance, even for one night, as worth the risk of HIV infection. Societal myths about HIV are reflected in unique ways within the transgender community. For example, some transsexuals believe that a change from a gay or lesbian to a heterosexual role, or a change from male to female, provides them with protection from HIV, without any concomitant behavior change. Moreover, the chronic lack of HIV prevention efforts targeting the transgender community has been seen as supporting a denial of risk already widespread in the community.

These and other transgender-specific HIV risks and prevention needs received national attention in 1995 during a community research development meeting held in conjunction with the Seventeenth National Lesbian and Gay Health Conference/Thirteenth Annual AIDS/HIV Forum. Hosted by the University of Minnesota Program in Human Sexuality, this meeting brought together community representatives, researchers, and funding agencies for the shared purpose of defining HIV prevention priorities. The transgender working group recommended that efforts be focused on building trust among communities, researchers, and policymakers; conducting multisite, epidemiological studies of HIV prevalence; developing prevention programming not limited to sex workers; empowering the transgender community; and fostering international collaboration.

The participation of transgenders in this meeting also exposed the limitations of existing HIV prevention and research in general. Such research typically has reflected conventional understandings of sex, gender, and sexual orientation, which in turn have defined established categories of risk and corresponding interventions. Transgenders challenge these categories, demonstrating that sex and gender are not binary, that sexual orientation and behavior are not synonymous, and that identities and behaviors are not static but may fluctuate over time and across situations. Understanding transgender identity and sexuality forces us to move beyond these limitations, to appreciate the context and complexity of HIV risk, and to develop more effective interventions for all.

Assessment of the needs of HIV-positive transgender persons revealed inadequate psychosocial support and a lack of knowledge and sensitivity on the part of health providers and prevention workers (Bockting, Robinson, and Rosser, 1998). The Gender Identity Support Services for Transgenders (1995)—a Boston-based project founded by transgender activist Rebecca Durkee—developed a curriculum and trained providers. The Harry Benjamin International Gender Dysphoria Association—a professional organization of providers and researchers—formed a task force on HIV/AIDS and surveyed gender clinics and surgeons regarding treatment services for HIV-positive transgenders (Avery, Cole, and Meyer, 1997). Findings showed little uniformity in how providers approach HIV-positive transgender clients. The Benjamin Association adopted the following resolution ensuring HIV-positive transgenders access to sex reassignment services: "The availability of sex reassignment surgery should not be denied solely on the basis of blood seropositivity for blood-borne infections (such as HIV, hepatitis B or C, etc.)" (Robinson, 1997, p. 2).

These efforts clearly signal that the silence once surrounding transgender and HIV has been broken. Here, we present reports on the first generation of transgender HIV prevention, research, and care initiatives. These reports were previously published online as a special issue of the *International Journal of Transgenderism* (Bockting and Kirk, 1999) and are reprinted with permission.

This compilation begins with a chapter by Inciardi, Surratt, Telles, and Pok, whose work with transvestite sex workers in Rio de Janeiro, Brazil, illustrates how marginalization impacts the effectiveness of HIV prevention programming. Their study of 100 *travestis* assessed HIV prevalence, drug use, and sexual behavior, revealing how idenity intersects with HIV risk. The authors argue that prevention efforts need to take into account participants' unique self-views and sexual roles, and that even though introduction of the female condom appeared promising, safer-sex instructions seem insufficient to address the complexity of *travestis'* HIV risk.

In Chapters 2 and 3, medical anthropologists Kammerer, Mason, and Connors and their collaborator Durkee discuss findings from their ethnographic research conducted in Boston, Massachusetts. Transgender people's difficulties with social affilations and their central struggle for social acceptance of who they are emerged as crucial factors placing transgenders at particular risk for HIV. The authors challenge the concept of "risk group" in understanding HIV risk, though they argue the importance in HIV prevention of fostering a group identity among transgenders. Further, they describe a lack of access to transgender-sensitive health and social services and outline common misperceptions among providers. They recommend that HIV prevention contribute to diminishing the social stigma that shapes both transgenders' HIV risk and their difficulties in obtaining appropriate services.

In Chapter 4, Reback and Lombardi report on the experience of serving transgenders in a community-based harm reduction program in Hollywood, California. The authors examined the role of sex work and substance abuse in HIV risk. Sex work was associated with greater substance use and greater numbers of both exchange and nonexchange sexual partners, but also with higher use of condoms. Thus, the authors conclude that in their sample, the sexual HIV risk of sex workers may be lower than that of non-sex workers. They recommend that future studies explore how the legal, social, and eco-

nomic situations of transgender persons contribute to marginalization and participation in sex work.

In Chapter 5, Clements-Nolle, Wilkinson, Kitano, and Marx present their assessment of the level of HIV risk behaviors and access to
services among transgenders in San Francisco. Unprotected sex, sex
work, and injection drug use were common. The authors identified
multiple barriers that transgender people face in accessing HIV prevention and health services. High levels of unemployment and homelessness demonstrate the need for job training, education, and housing placement. Participants in this study called for the hiring of
transgender persons to develop and implement targeted health and
social services.

As part of a larger study in Quebec, Canada, Namaste identifies salient issues for female-to-males in Chapter 6. These issues include a
lack of educational materials accounting for their bodies and sexualities, denial of risk, poor access to needles for hormone injection, low
self-esteem, and administrative practices that exclude female-to-males
from social services. Namaste challenges us to consider how sociopolitical factors contribute to transgenders' vulnerability to HIV infection. Moreover, she explains how research can facilitate social integration of transgenders through active involvement and collaboration.

In Chapter 7, Hein and Kirk present the results of their collaboration in offering a series of HIV prevention workshops for Enterprise,
a support group for female-to-male transsexuals of different sexual
orientations and different stages of gender transition in Greater Boston.
Going beyond information-based strategies, their approach uncov-
ered psychosocial and sexual issues of participants. Participants explored the roles and meanings of particular sexual behaviors in the
context of their identity development. The workshops therefore focused as much on sexual health as on HIV prevention.

In Chapter 8, Bockting, Rosser, and Coleman discuss the process
of bringing together various segments of the transgender community
in Minneapolis-St. Paul, to develop targeted HIV prevention education. Community members were actively involved in every aspect of
the program. The community's distrust of researchers, practitioners,
and policymakers surfaced, but working through the associated conflicts ultimately deepened mutual respect and solidified future collaboration. This chapter illustrates how university-based gender programs
can facilitate community building and empowerment.

In Chapter 9, Warren reviews the HIV prevention efforts of the Gender Identity Project in New York City, a peer-driven project that relies on transgender people to help one another assess community needs and create support mechanisms. The Project produced a video focusing on HIV prevention in the context of community building that features transgender and transexual persons, cross-dressers, and drag queens talking frankly about their transgender-specific HIV risks. Other prevention strategies described in this chapter include a multicultural and multi-identity peer outreach and education team, tailored safer-sex kits, and services that address psychosocial issues affecting HIV risk.

In Chapter 10, Wilson reports on his findings in performing sex reassignment surgery for HIV-positive transsexuals in Detroit. Wilson has provided this service since 1988 when the ethics committees of the two medical centers in which he operates deemed it unethical to withhold surgery because of HIV positivity alone.

In the final chapter, Kirk provides recommended guidelines for selecting and preparing HIV-positive patients for genital reconstructive surgery. She discusses how to manage these patients postoperatively and describes her experience with implementing these guidelines in her practice in Pittsburgh.

Together, these reports reflect the gap between the extent to which the HIV/AIDS epidemic has affected the transgender community and the availability of appropriate prevention and care services. The social stigma transgender people face compounds their HIV risk through neglect, low self-esteem, hunger for validation, rejection, employment discrimination, and disenfranchisement. At this time, we do not have an adequate response to the enormity of this problem. On the positive side, the transgender community has been able to mobilize and empower itself and has found a voice that no longer can be ignored. Transgender HIV prevention services now exist and are growing in number. Health professionals are becoming more aware and knowledgeable about the needs of their transgender clients. Transgender HIV prevention research contributes to a deeper understanding of the context of HIV risk. We call on transgender and nontransgender people alike to work together to advance HIV prevention and to promote our sexual health.

Walter Bockting
Sheila Kirk

REFERENCES

Avery, E.N., Cole, C.M., and Meyer, W.J., III (1997). "A Survey of gender clinics and surgeons regarding current treatment services for HIV+ transgendered individuals." Paper presented at the XV Harry Benjamin International Gender Dysphoria Association Symposium, Vancouver, British Columbia, Canada, September 13.

Bockting, W.O. and Kirk, S. (1999). Transgender and HIV: Risks, prevention, and care. *International Journal of Transgenderism* [Online serial], 3(1/2). Available <www.symposion.com/ijt/>.

Bockting, W.O., Robinson, B.E., and Rosser, B.R.S. (1998). Transgender HIV prevention: A qualitative needs assessment. *AIDS Care,* 10(4), 505-526.

Gender Identity Support Services for Transgenders (1995). *The invisible community: Transgenders and HIV risks: Training curriculum.* Boston, MA: Beacon Hill Multicultural Psychological Association.

Minnesota Department of Health (1994). *Minnesota comprehensive HIV/STD prevention plan 1995-1996.* Minneapolis, MN: Minnesota Department of Health, AIDS/STD Prevention Services Section.

Robinson, B.E. (Ed.) (1997). HBIGDA resolutions. *The Harry Benjamin International Gender Dysphoria Association Newsletter,* 7(2), 2.

Chapter 1

Sex, Drugs, and the Culture
of *Travestismo* in Rio de Janeiro

James A. Inciardi
Hilary L. Surratt
Paulo R. Telles
Binh H. Pok

In Brazil, transvestism is a specific social and cultural construct in which both gender and sexuality are mapped out and performed in highly particular ways.[1] Moreover, it has a long history, both as an integral theme during Carnaval and as a gender variation with its own distinct culture.[2,3,4] At Carnaval, best described as an enthusiastically celebrated street festival and parade during the five days prior to Ash Wednesday, many males—both gay and heterosexual—participate dressed as women, not only to glorify and venerate women, but also as a projection of male sexual fantasies.[5]

In contrast to Carnaval cross-dressing, the *travestis* of Brazil view transvestism as an identity and a designation that pervades every aspect of their lives. Although the clinical literature emphasizes that transvestites do not live continuously in the cross-gender role, and that their cross-dressing is periodic and fetishistic,[6,7] for the *travestis* of Brazil, transvestism appears to be enduring—typically lifelong.

This research was supported by NIH Grant No. UO1-DA08510, "HIV/AIDS Community Outreach in Rio de Janeiro, Brazil," from the National Institute on Drug Abuse. Correspondence and requests for materials should be sent to James A. Inciardi, PhD, Center for Drug and Alcohol Studies, University of Delaware, 77 East Main Street, Newark, DE 19716; Tel: (302) 831-6286; Fax: (302) 831-1275; e-mail: <jainyc@aol.com>.

Transvestites in Brazil, as in other cultures, are marked by an exaggerated femininity in both dress and makeup. They come almost exclusively from the poorest segments of Brazilian society, but there is little toleration for them in either the *favelas* (shantytowns) or the traditional, low-income suburban areas. Thus, as they begin to cross the lines of gender, most leave behind family and friends, emigrating to Rio de Janeiro, São Paulo, and other large cities, into districts where

> a mixture of socially marginal and often illegal activities creates not only a kind of moral region but a moral anonymity in which the traditional values of Brazilian society cease to function. Within this world (which is also the world of female prostitution, drug trafficking, homosexuality, and the more sporadic prostitution of the *miches* [male prostitutes]), given pervasive prejudice and discrimination, almost no options other than prostitution are open to the *travesti* for earning a living; as a result, almost all *travestis* quickly become involved in prostitution as their primary activity.[8]

Most transvestites live in close proximity to one another, and they always dress as women. Many use drugs, and because of their involvement in street prostitution, they are regularly exposed to both violence and a full range of sexually transmitted diseases, including HIV and AIDS. For example, among fifty-seven drug-using transvestites engaging in prostitution in Rome (the great majority of whom had emigrated from Brazil), the overall prevalence of HIV was 74 percent.[9] Studies conducted in various parts of Brazil over the past ten years also reflect high rates of HIV seropositivity among transvestite sex workers. Among thirty-seven transvestites tested in São Paulo during 1988, 62 percent were found to be HIV positive,[10] and among 112 transvestites contacted four years later, 60.7 percent tested positive.[11] Rio de Janeiro has, at least, an estimated 2,000 transvestites (and they prefer the term "transvestite," or *travesti* in Brazilian Portuguese, as opposed to transsexual or transgender), 80 percent of whom support themselves through prostitution. Within this context, the following discussion examines aspects of the subculture of male transvestite sex workers in Rio de Janeiro, with a particular focus on their drug-using and sexual risk behaviors.

METHODS

The data reported here were collected as part of a larger HIV/AIDS prevention initiative funded by the National Institute on Drug Abuse. Known as PROVIVA (Projeto Venha Informar-se sobre o Virus da AIDS) [Project Informing You About the AIDS Virus], the project operated between 1993 and 1997 as a collaborative effort between the University of Miami School of Medicine and the State University of Rio de Janeiro. Its general purposes were to establish a community-based HIV/AIDS surveillance and monitoring system and to develop and evaluate a culturally appropriate prevention-intervention program for cocaine users in Rio's *favelas* and red-light districts. A total of 1,643 individuals were recruited into the project, of whom 100 were male transvestite sex workers.

Data collection on these *travestis* occurred in two phases: (1) street recruitment as part of the overall project outreach and intervention effort and (2) focus groups.

Two cohorts of male transvestite prostitutes were sampled for this study. The first (N = 52) were recruited from the "Lapa" and "Copacabana" neighborhoods of Rio de Janeiro. Lapa is a downtown section of the city described in the guidebooks as an inner residential area, with some sections having numerous strip clubs and cheap hotels, many of which are considered "hot pillow establishments."[12,13] It is an old Bohemian area, famous in the past for its night life. However, as drug users, prostitutes, and transvestites began moving into Lapa and establishing themselves, the area began to deteriorate. Late at night, along such thoroughfares as Mem de Sá and Riachuelo, transvestite prostitutes in various states of undress can be observed soliciting their clientele.

Copacabana, famous since the 1920s as a flamboyant ocean resort, is a narrow, curving expanse covering just over four square kilometers. It is the most populous community in Rio de Janeiro, and its 250,000 residents make it one of the most densely inhabited areas of the world. High-rise apartments and hotels line the elite and expensive beachfront Avenida Atlântica, but behind it are 109 narrow streets and alleyways that mark a neighborhood in which as many as ten people are often crammed into small, two-bedroom apartments. Although prostitutes are active on many streets in Copacabana, including "Posto 6" and Rua Rainha Elizabeth, late at night transvestites can be found concentrated on an easterly segment of Avenida Atlântica, not too distant from the world-renowned, five-star Hotel Meridien.

The second cohort (N = 48) was sampled from a distant suburb of Rio de Janeiro known as Baixada Fluminense, an area containing more than 2.6 million people, the majority of whom are living in abject poverty. The Baixada is considered one of the poorest areas of Brazil, with infant mortality rates and incidence of infectious diseases five times higher than in Rio de Janeiro. Lacking a sewerage disposal system and potable drinking water, and awash in garbage, Baixada Fluminense is considered a public health disaster where tetanus, typhoid, meningitis, and a variety of intestinal infections are commonplace, especially among children.[14] Yet, surprisingly, rates of HIV infection tend to be lower in the Baixada than in the downtown sections of Rio de Janeiro.[15]

Initially, the recruitment of male transvestite sex workers for PROVIVA was conducted by outreach workers, on a one-night-a-week basis. Because transvestites are highly reviled in Rio de Janeiro and are frequently the targets of violence, outreach workers typically operated in pairs for the sake of their own personal safety. Contacts were made on the street and in the bars, strip clubs, hotels, and rooming houses frequented by transvestites. Success at recruitment was limited, however, for a variety of reasons. First, the great majority of the transvestites contacted began "working" quite late in the night and slept most of the day, and consequently, they were unwilling to visit PROVIVA during the project's operating hours. Second, the travel stipend paid to PROVIVA clients was R$10 in Brazilian currency (about U.S.$10 at the time the project was conducted) for each visit and was considered too low to entice many transvestite sex workers to make the trip. For those coming from Baixada Fluminense, the commute was nearly two hours by bus. Third, many were either afraid of being tested for HIV or already knew their HIV status. Finally, because of widespread discrimination against transvestites, many were suspicious of any university-based project, including PROVIVA.

As an alternative to traditional outreach techniques, two additional procedures were implemented. Since the latex condoms available in Rio de Janeiro are expensive and sometimes of low quality, transvestite recruits were promised forty U.S.-made condoms in addition to the regular travel stipend when they appeared at the PROVIVA office. Moreover, transvestite key informants from local organizations were retained as part-time outreach workers to increase the rapport between the project and the client population. These key informants were enthusiastic about working for the project because it targeted members of their peer group who were in great need of HIV prevention information. The new strategies resulted in the recruitment of fifty-two transvestite sex workers from Lapa and Copacabana, and forty-eight from Baixada Fluminense.

Once contacted in the field, all project clients were either transported or given directions to the PROVIVA assessment center, located in the São Cristóvão section of Rio de Janeiro. Interviewing, drawing of blood for HIV testing, pre- and posttest counseling, and AIDS prevention training were conducted at this center. Intake included informed consent, drug testing, and administration of a standardized Risk Behavior Assessment (RBA) interview instrument. Individual pretest HIV prevention counseling was provided, covering such topics as HIV disease, transmission routes, risky behaviors, risks associated with crack or cocaine use, rehearsal of male and female condom use, stopping unsafe sex practices, communication with partners, cleaning and disinfection of injection equipment, rehearsal of needle and syringe cleaning, disposal of hazardous waste material, stopping unsafe drug use, and the benefits of drug treatment. Voluntary HIV testing, distribution of relevant literature, and treatment referrals were also done at intake. An effort was made to reassess all participants at a follow-up session three to five months later, with a standardized Risk Behavior Follow-Up Assessment (RBFA) interview instrument, followed by HIV retesting and counseling for previously seronegative clients.

Descriptive statistics were compiled on demographic characteristics, drug use, and sexual behaviors of the participants. Multivariate logistic regression analyses were then conducted to examine the relationship between HIV seropositivity and its predictors. The independent variables entered into the model included age, race/ethnicity, level of education, income, sample, history of cocaine use, history of injection drug use, history of trading sex for drugs, Sexually Transmitted Disease (STD) history, number of sexual partners in the past thirty days, unprotected receptive anal sex in the past thirty days, unprotected insertive anal sex in the past thirty days, cocaine use during sex, and previous access to risk reduction information.

FINDINGS

Because the lifestyles and patterns of sexual behavior appear to be similar among both samples of the male transvestite sex workers recruited into this study, the data for each of the two cohorts are presented aggregately. As illustrated in Table 1.1, the transvestites sampled were young, with a median age of twenty-six years. The overwhelming majority had minimal education, with only 22 percent completing more than eight years of school. Further, white, black (Afro-Brazilian), and multiracial (mulato, pardo, and moreno) individuals were evenly represented in the sample. The data in Table 1.1 also suggest that the earnings of these transvestites were not high.

TABLE 1.1. Demographic Characteristics of 100 Male Transvestite Sex Workers, Rio de Janeiro, Brazil

Age at Interview	Percentage of Sample
18-24	34.0
25-34	51.0
35+	15.0
(Median age = 26)	
Race/Ethnicity	
Black	32.0
White	38.0
Multiracial	30.0
Education	
Less than 8 years	78.0
More than 8 years	22.0
Monthly Income*	
Less than $100	16.0
$101-$300	32.0
$301-$600	29.0
$601-$1,000	14.0
$1,001+	7.0
Don't know	2.0

*Income data were collected as number of minimum wages, then converted into U.S. dollars using an average minimum salary of R$100 per month at an exchange rate of 1:1 at the time the project was conducted.

The median monthly income of the sample was U.S.$450.00, which is equivalent to the salary of a part-time secretary or a research interviewer in Brazil. Also, although the data are not delineated in Table 1.1, four-fifths of the sample reported earnings through prostitution during the thirty-day period prior to interview, with the remaining 20 percent having income from other illegal activities, selling/trading goods, odd jobs, and/or friends and relatives.

Table 1.2 indicates that almost all of the transvestites had histories of alcohol use (91 percent), and that the majority had some experience with both marijuana (61 percent) and cocaine (76 percent). Other drugs, such as heroin, amphetamines, and hallucinogens are not listed because they are generally unavailable in Rio de Janeiro. In

TABLE 1.2. Drug Use Histories of 100 Male Transvestite Sex Workers, Rio de Janeiro, Brazil

Substance	Percent Ever Using
Alcohol	91.0
Marijuana	61.0
Cocaine	76.0
	Median Age at First Use
Alcohol	15.0
Marijuana	22.0
Cocaine	20.0
	Percent Using in Last 30 Days
Alcohol	68.0
Marijuana	26.0
Cocaine	55.0
Percent Ever Injecting Drugs	12.0
Percent Ever in Drug Treatment	5.0

terms of sequential patterns of drug use onset, the first drug used was alcohol at a median age of fifteen years, followed by cocaine and marijuana. During the thirty-day period prior to being enrolled into the project, 68 percent reported alcohol use, 26 percent reported marijuana use, and 55 percent reported cocaine use. Finally, only 12 percent reported any injection drug use, and even fewer (5 percent) had had any treatment for substance abuse.

Because the male transvestites contacted as part of this project were active sex workers, sexual risk behaviors were not uncommon. As illustrated in Table 1.3, most had numerous sex partners in the month prior to interview, and 50 percent reported engaging in sex with at least thirty different partners. Significant proportions also reported histories of sexually transmitted diseases, participation in both receptive and insertive anal sex, exchanging sex for drugs, and sex while under the influence of cocaine.

Of the 100 male transvestite sex workers studied in this prevention-intervention program, 48 percent tested positive for antibodies to HIV. As indicated in Table 1.4, multivariate logistic regression analyses found that the risk factors significantly related to HIV seropositivity included older age, lower education, having ever injected

TABLE 1.3. Sexual Behavior of 100 Male Transvestite Sex Workers, Rio de Janeiro, Brazil

Number of Sexual Partners*	Percentage of Sample
Fewer than 10	34.0
10-30	16.0
31+	50.0
Unprotected Insertive Anal Sex*	13.0
Unprotected Receptive Anal Sex*	32.0
Cocaine Use During Sex*	31.0
Ever Traded Sex for Drugs	29.0
STD History	39.0

*Reference period is thirty days prior to interview.

TABLE 1.4. Significant Predictors of HIV Infection for 100 Male Transvestite Sex Workers, Rio de Janeiro, Brazil

	Regression Coefficient	Odds Ratio	95% CI (Confidence Interval)
Sample*	− 2.128	.119	(.03, 43)
Age*	1.661	5.267	(1.51, 18.3)
Education*	− 1.750	.174	(.04, .81)
Drug Injection History*	2.458	11.682	(1.07, 128.12)
Unprotected Insertive Anal Sex*	2.160	8.670	(1.21, 62.2)

*Reference category for sample is sample 1; reference category for age is 25 or less; reference category for education is less than 8 years of school; reference category for injection history is no; reference category for unprotected insertive anal sex is no.

drugs, and having had unprotected insertive anal sex. Surprisingly, none of the other variables in the model, including unprotected receptive anal sex, appeared to relate to serostatus.

Because this project counted among its aims the reassessment of HIV risk behavior levels among clients who participated in the intervention, an attempt was made to recontact the 100 participants three months after the baseline interview. Because the recruitment difficulties noted earlier in this chapter persisted in the follow-up phase of the project, only thirty-nine of the participants who were contacted agreed to be reinterviewed. When examining risk behaviors at follow-up, no changes were apparent on any of the sexual behavior dimensions. In other words, participants neither decreased the number of sexual partners, modified the types of sexual activities engaged in, nor increased condom use in response to the intervention.

Given that the male transvestites contacted as part of the PROVIVA project were active sex workers, exchanged sex for drugs and/or money, had numerous sex partners, had histories of sexually transmitted diseases, and participated in both receptive and insertive anal sex, it is not surprising that almost half tested positive for antibodies to HIV. However, because the RBA was a standardized instrument designed primarily for injection drug users, few questions related to historical sexual risks, and none of the questions targeted the special risks associated with male transvestite sex work. Furthermore, the RBA had not been designed to elicit information about cultural and lifestyle issues. As a result, the investigators conducted seven focus groups, each containing five to eight transvestites. Topics included their views of prostitution and transvestism, employment patterns, sexual activities, condom use, drug use, and mechanisms of feminization.

During these sessions participants described the feminization process using silicone, a virtually unstudied potential risk factor for HIV transmission among male transvestites.[16] The focus group data suggested that the use of silicone was widespread among the 100 clients recruited into the project. It was reported that the great majority of the transvestites in Rio undergo silicone injections to shape their bodies. These "beauty treatments," as the clients referred to them, were done by other "experienced" transvestites who are too old to support themselves as street prostitutes. The injection equipment was typically shared by several transvestites, with less than adequate cleaning between each use. Industrial quality silicone was most commonly used because it could be purchased by the gallon at a relatively low price. Numerous injections, sometimes more than seventy punctures, were required to accomplish each individual body shape. Since this was a painful process, it was common for transvestites to be under the influence of alcohol and/or drugs during the process. The injected liquid silicone had a tendency to dislodge after a few months, and, thus, new injections were required periodically to reshape certain parts of the body. Moreover, infections were common after such procedures, and often plastic surgery was the only recourse to remove the dislodged silicone.

The general lack of insight into the role of the *travestis* as they define it further attests to the marginalization of the population. For example, focus group data indicate that the *travestis* of Rio de Janeiro, contrary to much of the literature on transvestism, do not consider themselves to be heterosexual. Although they report feeling sexually attracted to men, they do not identify themselves as either women or male homosexuals. Rather, they view themselves as having a separate gender identity, which they designate as "transvestite." Furthermore, unlike gay men, transvestites do not have a sexual interest in male homosexuals, but in men "who are normally attracted to women."

Ideally, the *travestis* wish their sex partners to look at them as women, to take the active role in anal intercourse, and to ignore the transvestite's masculine genitalia during sex. A transvestite typically keeps "her" penis hidden from her insertive partners during sexual intercourse through special clothes or posture. However, this act of "hiding" is more apt to take place when a transvestite sex worker is engaging in sexual activity with clients as opposed to her steady partner. Playing the active role in a sexual encounter is considered by many participants to be a violation of their "ideal sexuality," although many engaged in this behavior to satisfy their clientele.

Although transvestites dress and make themselves up as women, it is not their intent to "pass" as women. The ideal expressed by transvestites is to perform the traditional gender roles of women—being a wife and a homemaker and cooking for the partner—without physically becoming women. In fact, many voiced a special repugnance for the vagina and considered transsexual surgery to be nonsensical. These attitudes were a reflection of two convictions held strongly by this group of transvestites: On the one hand, they tended to devalue women as a group, and the vagina was a symbol of being biologically female. At the same time, the transvestites considered themselves to possess a separate, special kind of sexual identity in which the ideal of the feminine role is achieved without requiring the full female anatomy.

DISCUSSION

The high rate of HIV infection observed among male transvestite sex workers demonstrates the need to include this population in both outreach and intervention efforts. Yet this Rio-based initiative failed to demonstrate any significant behavioral changes subsequent to the intervention. This, however, was not surprising to the investigators, since the standardized intervention utilized had been designed for primarily drug-using populations. In fact, the purpose of the pilot study among the *travestis* was to better understand the unique HIV/AIDS and special needs of Brazilian transvestite sex workers.

An effective AIDS prevention initiative targeting this population must take these notions of gender identity and sexuality into account and include the following strategies. First, although transvestite sex workers are aware of the importance of condoms during anal sex, few actually use them. Not only are condoms expensive, but the transvestites' clients are often unwilling to use them. As such, not only must there be greater availability of condoms, but also mechanisms to teach transvestites how to negotiate condom use with clients. Condom negotiation and empowerment techniques have long been a part of risk reduction initiatives for women, but because transvestites are typically looked upon as "men," this aspect of prevention programming is typically forgotten.

Second, the investigators were the first to introduce the female condom to Brazilian transvestites.[17,18] Pilot work determined that, not only did transvestite sex workers consider the female condom to be an acceptable method of HIV risk reduction during anal sex, but also that they liked it and were willing and eager to use it. As such, female condom distribution and instruction in its use would appear to be a crucial part of AIDS prevention for this population.

Third, there is the problem of the repeated use of contaminated needles and syringes during silicone injections. This is not a topic that is addressed in contemporary AIDS prevention programs. Although the cleaning of injection paraphernalia is discussed with drug users, more general HIV prevention discussions bypass the topic. In this regard, information about the hazards associated with using potentially infected needles must be provided not only to transvestite sex workers but also to the other members of their subculture who actually administer the injections.

NOTES

1. Parker, R.G. (1989). "Youth, Identity, and Homosexuality: The Changing Shape of Sexual Life in Brazil," *Journal of Homosexuality* 17:269-289.

2. Bloom, P. (1997). *Brazil Up Close* (Edison, NJ: Hunter).

3. Linger, D.T. (1992). *Dangerous Encounters: Meaning of Violence in a Brazilian City* (Stanford, CA: Stanford University Press).

4. Scheper-Hughes, N. (1992). *Death Without Weeping: The Violence of Everyday Life in Brazil* (Berkeley: University of California Press).

5. *Manchete* 46, February 15, 1997.

6. Docter, R.F. (1988). *Transvestites and Transsexuals: Toward a Theory of Cross-Gender Behavior* (New York: Plenum Press).

7. Docter, R.F. and V. Prince (1997). "Transvestism: A Survey of 1032 Cross Dressers," *Archives of Sexual Behavior* 26:589-605.

8. Daniel, H. and R.G. Parker (1993). *Sexuality, Politics, and AIDS in Brazil* (London: Falmer Press), p. 91.

9. Gattari, P., L. Spizzichino, C. Valenzi, M. Zaccarelli, and G. Rezza (1992). "Behavioural Patterns and HIV Infection Among Drug Using Transvestites Practicing Prostitution in Rome," *AIDS Care* 4:83-87.

10. Suleiman J., G. Suleiman, and G.P.A. Ayroza (1989). "Seroprevalence of HIV Among Transvestites in the City of São Paulo." Paper presented at the V International Conference on AIDS, Montreal, June 4-9.

11. Grandi, J.L., A.C. Ferreira, and A. Kalichman (1993). "HIV and Syphilis Infection Among Transvestites in São Paulo City." Paper presented at the IX International Conference on AIDS, Berlin, June 6-11.

12. Box, B. (1994). *South American Handbook* Seventieth (70th) Edition. Chicago: NTC Publishing Group.

13. Box, B. (1997). *South American Handbook* Seventy-third Edition. Chicago: NTC Publishing Group.

14. Taylor, E. (1994). *Rio de Janeiro* (Boston: Houghton-Mifflin).

15. Telles, P.R., H.L. Surratt, and J.A. Inciardi (1996). "Assessing the Regional Distribution of HIV Prevalence Among Drug Users in Rio de Janeiro." Paper presented at the XI International Conference on AIDS, Vancouver, British Columbia, Canada, July 7-12.

16. Goihman S., A. Ferreira, S. Santos, and J.L. Grandi (1994). "Silicone Application As a Risk Factor for HIV Infection." Paper presented at the X International Conference on AIDS, Yokohama, Japan, August 7-12.

17. Inciardi, J.A. and H.L. Surratt (1995). "The Use of the Female Condom for Anal Sex." Paper presented at the III National Conference of Transvestites and the Liberated, Rio de Janeiro, Brazil, June 13-16.

18. Inciardi, J.A. and H.L. Surratt (1996). "The Female Condom and the Prevention of AIDS." Paper presented at the International Forum on the Prevention of Drug Use and AIDS, Institute for the Development of the Amazon, Belem, Brazil, April 19.

Chapter 2

Transgenders, HIV/AIDS, and Substance Abuse: From Risk Group to Group Prevention

Nina Kammerer
Theresa Mason
Margaret Connors
Rebecca Durkee

In 1995, three of the authors undertook anthropological research in partnership with the fourth, Rebecca Durkee, the founder of a community-based transgender organization in Boston, Massachusetts. Gender Identity Support Services for Transgenders (GISST) addresses the health and community needs of transgenders and transsexuals, particularly the most economically and psychologically vulnerable male-to-females, many of whom engage in prostitution and substance abuse.[1] In this chapter, transgender is used inclusively as encompassing transsexual.

The authors acknowledge funding from the Massachusetts Department of Public Health, HIV/AIDS Bureau that supported the research on the AIDS prevention and care needs of Boston's transgender community from which the chapter draws. Our research would have been impossible without the cooperation of the many individuals who agreed to be interviewed or to participate in focus groups. This chapter builds on sections of *Transgenders and HIV Risk: Needs Assessment* (Mason, Connors, and Kammerer, 1995). We are grateful to Lee Strunin for including us on a panel she organized for the 1997 annual meeting of the Society for Applied Anthropology, at which an earlier version was presented, and to Stephen Koester, a panel discussant, for his encouraging comments. We are all deeply indebted to the many scholars and activists who have critiqued the HIV risk group model. Finally, we would like to thank our editors, Drs. Walter Bockting and Sheila Kirk, for including this chapter even though it was not part of the special journal issue on which this book is based.

GISST obtained funding from the Massachusetts Department of Public Health, HIV/AIDS Bureau to conduct an HIV/AIDS needs assessment for the transgenders it serves.[2] From April to August 1995, Theresa Mason, Margaret Connors, and Nina Kammerer conducted ethnographic field research and reviewed existing literature to understand what factors contribute to HIVrisk among transgenders and transsexuals in the Boston area. We included interviews with health and social service providers to explore their perceptions of, and responses to, transgendered people.

Our analysis of data from that research (Mason, Connors, and Kammerer, 1995) highlighted the relationship between the process of social marginalization and enhanced risk for HIV. The loss of status and often the related loss of economic security for genetic males who identify, and to varying degrees live, as females heighten their vulnerability. Their experiences provide further evidence for the ways that culturally defined power imbalances structure individuals' risk for HIV. In this chapter, we argue that these observations—based on ethnographic attentiveness to the way people describe their own personal histories—can shed light on epidemiological findings. They also indicate some limitations of epidemiologists' tendencies to operationalize social conditions as variables of group affiliation, as in "risk group." As we will describe, the crucial factors that place transgenders at particular risk for HIV and other sexually transmitted infections (STIs) are their very difficulties with social affiliations and their central struggle for social acceptance of who they are. We suggest alternative concepts for thinking about risk, specifically notions of historical and contemporary risk structures, to encourage movement away from overly concrete thinking—however implicit—about risk situations as social groups.

Two aspects of the relationship between ethnographic research on HIV risk factors and the epidemiology of HIV/AIDS merit mention. Ethnography (the practice of and knowledge from participant observation research) and epidemiology (the study of the distribution and determinants of disease) inevitably intersect in discussions of prevention strategies. This is because epidemiological research has exerted a major influence on prevention throughout the epidemic by defining who is targeted for prevention and how the movement of the epidemic is envisioned socially (Mann, 1993, 1999). As a result, the underlying assumptions and social implications of epidemiological concepts such as risk groups (or in more recent usage, transmission categories) raise methodological and conceptual issues for ethnographers (Kane and

Mason, 1992). Hence, our research, which was primarily intended to inform public health prevention work, also contributes to the social scientific critique of analyzing risk either through behavioral and psychological characteristics of individuals or through concepts that imply groups.

It is important, however, to keep in mind that concepts such as "group"—which are misleading in the *analysis* of what contributes to risk—are often important in the design of prevention *strategies.* Indeed, much HIV risk reduction programming can be characterized as efforts to create a sense of community and social support among peers for people who have been marginalized or alienated for a variety of reasons and therefore suffer from a lack of positive social affiliation. In this chapter, we argue that for transgendered people, as for others, group models confuse analyses of risk. At the same time, programs that encourage shared identity and collective action advance the goals of HIV/AIDS prevention campaigns.

After discussing the category of transgenders, we turn to the HIV/AIDS and related substance abuse risks of highly vulnerable male-to-female transgenders. Next we present a developmental and interactional model of HIV/AIDS and substance abuse risks among people served by GISST during the period of our research. We then examine what the social category of transgender reveals about the epidemiological risk group model, including what we label "the fallacy of misplaced groupness." In conclusion, we present an identity-based group model of prevention exemplified in efforts by Rebecca Durkee and other activists to build self-affirming social identities among transgenders.

TRANSGENDERS: UNDERSTANDINGS AND MISUNDERSTANDINGS

HIV/AIDS risks of transgenders cannot be comprehended without considering who belongs in this category, either through self-identity or through identification by others. Transsexuals and transgenders are now culturally hot in the United States, as evidenced by 1997 and 2000 Super Bowl advertisements that featured transgendered characters,[3] Leslie Feinberg's (1996) widely reviewed book *Transgender Warriors,* and depictions of transgendered individuals in media—the recent film *Boys Don't Cry* (1999) is one among many examples.

Nonetheless, despite their current cultural currency, the categories of transsexual and transgender are not well understood.

Transsexualism is often misidentified as having to do with sexual orientation rather than gender identity. This may be in part because of the label itself, which contains the word "sexual" (Stuart, 1991, p. 25). Yet there are heterosexual, homosexual, and bisexual transsexuals, whether by sexual behavior, orientation, or self-identity. The label transsexual, an older term than transgender, derives from medical science and reflects the more general cultural equation of gender and genitalia. Although sex reassignment surgery was first performed either in the 1920s (Bolin, 1994, p. 455) or 1930s (Raymond, 1994 [1979], p. 21), it did not begin to be well known or widely practiced until the 1950s, when the term transsexualism was coined and George Jorgenson became the famous Christine. In the United States, the Harry Benjamin Foundation was established in 1964, and the Johns Hopkins Gender Identity Clinic three years later (Raymond, 1994 [1979], pp. 21-22); the first male-to-female sex change operation was performed in 1965 (Stuart, 1991, p. 42). The Harry Benjamin Standards of Care, which define eligibility criteria for genital reconstructive surgery, are still influential in the field.

It is important to note that this view of transsexualism suggests that it is a psychopathological state. Transsexualism, also called gender dysphoria by medical and psychological specialists (Denny, 1994, p. xxi), is categorized in the American Psychiatric Association's (1980, p. 261) *Diagnostic and Statistical Manual of Mental Disorders,* Third Edition (DSM-III) under Gender Identity Disorders, which are disorders marked by "an incongruence between anatomic sex and gender identity." In the DSM-II (pp. 261-262), transsexualism is defined as "a persistent sense," lasting a minimum of two years, "of discomfort and inappropriateness about one's anatomic sex and a persistent wish to be rid of one's genitals and to live as a member of the other sex." In the revised third edition (DSM-III-R) (American Psychiatric Association, 1987, p. 74), "anatomic sex" is changed to "assigned sex." Transsexualism does not appear in either the index or the text of *Diagnostic and Statistical Manual of Mental Disorders,* Fourth Edition (DSM-IV) (American Psychiatric Association, 1994), but Gender Identity Disorder does. This disorder requires for diagnosis evidence of "a strong and persistent cross-gender identification" (p. 532) and "persistent discomfort about one's assigned sex or a sense of the inappropriateness in the gender role of that sex" (p. 533). Unlike transsexualism, its necessary diagnostic criteria do not include the desired to be rid of one's genitals. Yet with or without the label transsexualism, the existential condition of cross-gender identity experienced by transgenders remains officially pathologized.

The terms "preop" and "postop"—before and after the surgical operation for sex reassignment—spring from the medical model of transsexualism or gender dysphoria. These labels, which are used by transsexuals themselves, appear in escort advertisements in periodicals such as the *Boston Phoenix* (1995, p. 13): "Come worship this sexy Pre-op," "beautiful Amer-Asian Post op," "You've seen the Pre(before) ops(operation). But I'm a Post(after) op. See the finished product." Whereas some who have undergone surgery continue to think of themselves as transsexual, others identify as neither postop nor transsexual. Their crossing complete, they simply identify as female (for male-to-female) or male (for female-to-male).[4]

Until recently, medical and psychological specialists, as well as many transsexuals themselves, commonly viewed transsexuals as individuals who either wanted to have surgery or had already had it. This view is culturally constructed by our anatomical or biological essentialism. Sex, as Shelly Errington (1990, p. 27) astutely notes, "is the gender system of the West." Yet transgenders and transsexuals, feminists, and others now critique biological reductionism and cultural isomorphism of sex and gender. Not everyone who considers herself or himself transsexual wants to have sex reassignment surgery. For someone to self-identify today as preop does not necessarily mean that she or he hopes to undergo surgery—the terminology lingers even as the categories change. An activist pointed out that, for some people, "maintaining the factory-supplied plumbing is important." A male-to-female interviewee explained:

> We have sex with men, but we don't consider ourselves gay. I live my life as a woman, dress like a woman, but I use what I have. . . . I enjoy what I have. I enjoy using it during intimacy. I don't have the desire for the operation.

This statement clearly shows the inadequacy of labels such as gay or homosexual and of the often-heard phrase "woman trapped in a man's body" for describing transsexuals and transgenders.

In its most inclusive sense, transgender is an umbrella term that one interviewee described as "all inclusive of everyone with a gender issue." It can encompass "gays, lesbians, bisexuals, and straights who exhibit any kind of dress and/or behavior interpreted as 'transgressing' [traditional] gender roles" (Raymond, 1994 [1979], p. xxv). This label can embrace queens, whether drag queens, street queens, or just queens; transvestites and cross-dressers, whether gay or straight; and transsexuals, whether preop, postop, or those who do not opt for a sex change operation.[5]

Used expansively, the term "transvestite" or "cross-dresser" can be applied to anyone who wears one or more items of clothing normally identified with people of the other gender.[6] Typically, however, this label is applied to persons of one sex, usually male, who wear a full set of clothing culturally associated with the other gender in order to present themselves as people of that other gender. Many male transvestites are heterosexually identified and married. From a medical perspective, a transvestite male engages in fetishistic cross-dressing, often for sexual pleasure. He "cross-dresses not for money, entertainment, politics, nor because he is convinced that he is really a woman. He does it from perceived need, often expressed as compulsion, and because he enjoys it" (Woodhouse, 1989, p. x). The line between transgender and transvestite is not always clear-cut. For example, Woodhouse (1989, pp. 44-46) presents the case of Anne, a transvestite turned transsexual, who underwent sex reassignment surgery after having lived for years as a married, self-identified transvestite.

Around the umbrella label of transgender, a self-conscious political community—"a grass-root movement called transgenderism" (Rothblatt, 1995, p. 16; see also Bolin, 1994)—has been developing since the 1980s. Kate Bornstein (1994) and other transgendered activists such as Leslie Feinberg (1996), Nancy Nangeroni (1995), and Martine Rothblatt (1995) criticize the Euro-American binary gender system and its premise that gender equals genitalia. Whereas the "trans" prefix used to mean "to cross," in the sense of mixing categories (the "wrong body" view) or changing categories (through surgery), it can now mean "to go beyond," in the sense of transforming the previously rigid sex/gender system. This change in terminology is reflected in the name for GISST, in which the "T" first stood for transsexuals but now stands for transgenders.

Not all who self-identify as transgender are equally political, and transgender politics is not uniform. Some individuals self-identify as both transsexual and transgender, using these labels more or less interchangeably, whereas others once saw themselves as transsexuals but now see themselves as transgenders, and still others self-identify as exclusively either one or the other. These labels, at least until the time of our research, have evolved along class lines. Many working-class individuals encountered in our research whom we would identify as transgender were unaware of the term. This is not to say that some politicized transgenders, Rebecca Durkee included, are not of working-class origin. Labels and identities have changed and will continue to change. What will remain constant, however, is that transsexuals and transgenders, whether through their politics or just by their existence, challenge this culture's dichotomous classification of sex and gender.

Transgenders make clear that while sex, gender, and sexual orientation are interrelated, they are also separate. Thus sex, which is given at birth, does not determine gender or sexual orientation; neither does gender determine sexual orientation, or vice versa. Sex, as one transgendered activist put it, "is plumbing; sex is between your legs." Generally, the determination of sex at birth is unproblematic: female for an infant with a vagina, male for an infant with a penis. A very small number of people, however, are born physiologically intersexed or hermaphroditic. Gender is an aspect of identity, of self. In the transgendered activist's words, it is "your sense of 'am I a male,' 'am I a female,' 'am I neither,' 'am I both.' That's between your ears." Sexual orientation has to do with desire and arousal. Are you attracted to someone male by sex, male by gender, female by sex, female by gender, or some combination thereof? The inadequacy of the labels heterosexual, bisexual, and homosexual is immediately apparent. What from an outsider's perspective is homosexuality may be heterosexuality from the point of view of the participants. Many male-to-female transgenders consider themselves to be having heterosexual sex when they have sex with men.

HIV/AIDS AND SUBSTANCE ABUSE RISKS

Accurate statistics on HIV infection and AIDS among transgenders in the Boston area are unavailable, but at a 1999 memorial service for transgenders, organized by Rebecca Durkee, approximately 100 of the 153 individuals being mourned had died of AIDS-related illness.[7] The individuals served by GISST are at high risk for engaging in prostitution, reasons for which will be detailed in the section on risk structures. What is important to note in this discussion of HIV/AIDS, alcohol, and drugs is our research finding that participation in prostitution often precipitates alcohol and drug abuse. Especially given the literature on crack cocaine (e.g., Carlson and Siegal, 1991), drug use is often seen as what propels people into selling their bodies—the sex-for-drugs connection. Our respondents affirmed that for many transgenders it is engaging in sex work that leads to abusing alcohol and/or drugs, not the other way around. Of course, alcohol and drug use can increase the risk of HIV infection already posed by participating in prostitution, as well as by engaging in unprotected noncommercial sex.

Although accurate statistics on transgenders' alcohol and drug use are scarce, substantial evidence in the published literature and from our interviews in the Boston area indicates that such use is widespread and significantly detrimental to their health. For example, 66 percent of male transvestite prostitutes—male-to-female transgenders in the terminology adopted here—in an Atlanta study used crack cocaine (Elifson et al., 1993, p. 261, Table 1), while another study in the same city found that 71 and 56.3 percent of those in two geographical areas used (Boles and Elifson, 1994, p. 89, Table 2).[8] Use of intravenous heroin has been reported, but no statistics are available. Both Rebecca Durkee and an interviewee estimated that at least 80 percent of Boston's transgenders have an alcohol and/or drug problem. For the transgenders served by GISST, alcohol use is encouraged simply because bars are the locus for socializing and for picking up tricks. Studies, especially of adolescents, have found an association between alcohol use and sexual behavior, particularly sexual risk behavior (e.g., Strunin and Hingson, 1992).

A drug risk unique to transgenders is injections of hormones obtained on the black market.[9] Hormones are shot intramuscularly rather than intravenously, but the reuse of unsterilized needles for intramuscular injections still poses an HIV risk (Packard and Epstein, 1992, p. 363).[10] We have been told of drag shows where all the performers who wanted hormones lined up and received them in turn from a single needle that was not cleansed between shots. These potent drugs are taken without assurance of quality, dosing prescription, or medical monitoring of effects. The accepted medical practice is to prescribe hormone pills to be taken orally, but many doctors prescribe intramuscular shots. Transgenders who either cannot afford to visit a doctor or do not meet the medical/psychological requirements to be diagnosed as transsexual turn to the black market to buy pills and/or injectable hormones, which are believed to be more effective. Male-to-female transgenders who do not have sex reassignment surgery must remain on high doses of female hormones to counteract their naturally produced testosterone.[11]

Our interviewees reported that they often take higher doses of hormones than are medically recommended to achieve a full and fast feminization. Even those taking hormones under a doctor's care may augment them from the black market to obtain this effect. One transgender described her attachment to the hormones that make her look and feel more feminine as being "addicted." Even transgenders whose hormone use is medically monitored report mood swings. Those whose use is subject to the vagaries of availability and ability to pay may experience more precipitate or acute swings. Such swings can prompt "acting out," in the words of transgenders, including risky behavior, whether involving sex or needles. Incarceration, a frequent consequence of engagement in prostitution and use of illegal drugs, results in the abrupt discontinuation of hormones. It does not, unfortunately, remove the risk of HIV infection, including through forced sex with guards or other inmates.

CONCEPTUALIZING RISK

Research by Boles and Elifson (1994, p. 85), among others, reported that "transvestite prostitutes"—transgendered prostitutes in the terminology adopted here—"have a high rate of HIV seropositivity relative to other sex workers." Despite the social science critiques, many epidemiologists and public health specialists are likely to interpret such findings as indications of yet another "risk group." Since, from an epidemiological point of view, small numbers do not justify creating an entirely new risk category, the search for an existing risk category in which to place transgendered people has been necessary. The tendency has been to place male-to-female transgenders in the "men who have sex with men" (MSM) risk category. MSM is a transformation of the Centers for Disease Control's original risk group for HIV—homosexuals—a change that acknowledged the diversity of sexual orientation identities among men who engage in sexual exchanges between men. Scholars and activists have pointed out the inadequacies of the risk group model (e.g., Connors, 1992; Kane and Mason, 1992; Oppenheimer, 1988, 1992; Schiller, 1992; Schiller,

Crystal, and Dewellen, 1994; Treichler, 1988, [1987]; Weeks, 1995). As Jeffrey Weeks (1995, p. 43) notes,

> The assumption that evidence of certain practices reveals the prevalence of identities is not only a fallacy, but a dangerous one, when it comes to health and safer-sex education, because it assumes that people will recognize themselves in social identities that are peculiar to very specific parts of the world.

The larger category of MSM was devised to capture all men who engage in sex with men, regardless of their sexual identity. As numerous authors have pointed out, many Latinos who have sex with other men do not self-identify as homosexual (Alonso and Koreck, 1990; Fry, 1985; Lancaster, 1995; Parker, 1985, 1989, 1991).[12] For them, what is culturally salient in defining masculinity is being the active rather than the passive partner in sexual intercourse.

As a transmission category, MSM is a more adequate descriptor than homosexual because it focuses on behavior, rather than identity. But this "well-intentioned label" (Weeks, 1995, p. 43), while avoiding the mistaken equation of sexual behavior with sexual orientation identity, conflates sexual biology and gender identity. The category MSM implicitly rests on our cultural reading of anatomy as identity, that to be born with a penis is to be a man. MSM does not accurately describe male-to-female transgenders who, although genetically male, experience a female gender identity. Prevention messages that target MSM leave out transgenders who consider themselves to be women— or neither men nor women—having sex with men—or with women or with both, depending on their sexual desires. Weeks (1995, p. 43) astutely observes that the move in AIDS prevention from homosexual to MSM "compounds the problem by offering a social position that no one recognizes themselves in." Whereas previous studies, by showing that homosexual sexual activity need not entail homosexual or gay identity, have deconstructed the equation of behavior and identity, the transgender case splits apart the identification of sexual anatomy with gender identity.

How then do we model transgenders' risks for HIV/AIDS and substance abuse? Instead of being viewed as a risk group, transgenders are better viewed as situated in what might be termed historical and contemporary risk structures. Although these structures are interconnected, their analytical separation can advance analysis of health risks and thereby inform prevention. Historical risk is longitudinal across the life cycle, whereas contemporary risk involves current social networks. The first is developmental, while the second is interactional, pertaining to ongoing social life.

Both historical and contemporary risk structures transcend the methodological individualism that pervades social scientific and public health research (Laumann and Gagnon, 1995, p. 206; see also Fee and Kreiger, 1993). Transgendered individuals are embedded in society and must be seen not as isolated actors but as people who interact in families, schools, and other social contexts. Risk structures allow for a shift in the analytical emphasis to include the reality and complexity of identities; the fluidity of social life; the power of cultural categories, meanings, and values; and the impact of stigma and discrimination.

The analytical use of the concept of historical risk structures turns attention to the experience, common among transgenders, of knowing themselves to be different from an early age, and to the stigma associated with that difference. Even before hearing labels such as transsexual and transgender, a transgendered child typically has a sense of self as different, as not fitting into the available categories. An interviewee in our study reported,

> This is something you become aware of at—pick a number—two, three, five, twelve. Some people say it's twenty or thirty, but I just don't believe that. And so you're a ten-year-old boy or . . . you're a five-year-old boy and you *know.* You know better than you know that the sun is going to come up tomorrow that this is something, this is the way you are, and it's fucked up.

When this interviewee said that her reality, realized at age three, was "fucked up," she meant that it transgressed society's dominant and dichotomous categories of sex and gender; she did not mean that it was psychopathological, as traditional psychiatry and society's standards would have it.

Many transgenders, including some of our interviewees, affirm that they knew their gender at a young age, whether as the opposite of biology (Bolin, 1988, p. 73; Stuart, 1991, pp. 40-41) or as neither boy nor girl, that is, what has come to be referred to as "non-traditional gender" (Bornstein, 1994, p. 8) or "third gender" (Herdt, 1994). They do not, however, affirm that they knew that others shared their difference. Indeed, many attest to learning only in adolescence or later that there were others similar to them. Thus, awareness of being different need not entail a distinct identity, much less one shared with others. Again, we can see that having attributes or displaying behaviors that others classify as belonging to a particular group does not mean that an individual identifies with that group. Someone can be trans-gendered without knowing that label or knowing that there is any other person who has experienced the same sense of difference from this culture's dichotomous classification of sex and gender.

As with historical risk structures, the concept of contemporary risk structures offers a more dynamic approach to analyzing risk. Fo-cusing on the kinds of contexts and specific settings where drug abuse and sexual exchanges are likely to occur provides a sense of the range of individuals who must be engaged in the risk reduction pro-cess. In downtown Boston, at the time of our research, two bars ca-tered to male-to-female transgenders and to men seeking their com-pany. Nontransgender patrons of these bars come from Boston and beyond. For example, we spoke with one married man in his thirties who regularly drives in from the suburbs to frequent one of these bars. The risk group paradigm leaves out such men and other drink-ing and sex partners of transgenders.

Clients of transgendered sex workers are often men who have un-resolved gender issues or have not come to terms with their sexual orientation. Transgendered sex workers report that their clients in-clude men who have not accepted their own homosexual desires and transvestites or cross-dressers—"Dressy Bessies," as they call them—who self-identify as straight. One transgendered sex worker said of her many clients, "It's not that they want a man and they want a woman. They're afraid of their sexuality, that they might be gay. So, if it's got a skirt on 'it,' it's okay!" (see also Bockting, Rosser, and Coleman, 1993, p. 29).

The complex identities of both transgenders and their sex partners call into question the epidemiological concept of "bridge," also re-ferred to as "bridge group" (Lima et al., 1994), "epidemic bridge" (Sankary et al., 1996), and "transmission bridge" (Wood, Rhodes, and Malotte, 1996). This concept, widespread in the contemporary biomedical and social scientific literature on HIV/AIDS, is predi-cated on the concept, already critiqued, of boundable groups. The concept of bridge also rests squarely on the notion of core groups or core transmitters, of which commercial sex workers are the prime exemplar. For example, a study "to determine the extent to which men provide a bridge population between commercial sex workers (CSW) and the general female population in Thailand" found that "[b]ridge populations may be as important as 'core groups' for the spread of HIV into the general Thai population" (Morris et al., 1996, p. 1265). It is but a short step from core groups and bridges to vectors. Indeed, one study of male street prostitutes in New Orleans calls these men not only "a bridge of HIV infection into populations with currently low infection rates" but also "a vector for the transmission of HIV infection into the heterosexual world" (Morse et al., 1991, p. 535)! Here we encounter what has been called "the third epidemic" of stigmatization and blame (Panos Institute, 1990).

Risk groups, core groups or core transmitters, and bridges all underplay the complexity of people's lives, identities, and behaviors. The image of a bridge evokes a connector between firm ground on two sides. When applied to people, it implies a linkage between one discrete group and another. The example of transgenders and their sex partners highlights the complexity of identities and interactions and the social, economic, and cultural construction of risk and risk taking. To view social network analysis as simply a better way of mapping "groups," as some researchers do (e.g., Rothenberg and Narramore, 1996), is to ignore the fundamental critique of group thinking that both the concept of network and the concept of risk structures entail.

BEYOND INDIVIDUAL AND PSYCHOLOGICAL RISK: HISTORICAL AND CONTEMPORARY RISK STRUCTURES

Our research found that precipitating factors for transgenders' sexual risks and substance abuse arise from three main sources: (1) social stigmatization and related negative self-image, (2) economic vulnerability and related prostitution and substance abuse, and (3) the need for identity affirmation and the quest for a feminine body.[13]

Social stigmatization is pivotal in transgenders' historical risk structures. The severe denial and denigration that transgenders face from childhood onward has been movingly depicted by Leslie Feinberg (1993) in her novel *Stone Butch Blues*. Because family, teachers, and friends deny their reality, which, as an interviewee cited earlier noted, is "fucked up" by society's standards, transgenders themselves become practiced in denial. This same interviewee observed, "Their greatest skill, the thing in which they are better than anybody in the universe, is denial." Indeed, "Queen of Denial" is a phrase used often by transgenders to describe themselves or their transgendered sisters.

Certainly, there are psychological dimensions to transgender risks for STIs and substance abuse, but these must be seen as forged by society. For some transgenders, societal pressures to conform to accepted gender norms and to hide their true identities, along with practical problems in realizing their desire or need to live as women, can lead to cycles of withdrawal and "acting out." Such cycles are often not conducive to tempered alcohol consumption, needle cleansing, or safer-sex practices. These psychological dimensions of risk must be understood as a function of the internalization of society's judgment. The negative self-image so common among transgenders is such an internalization, not a symptom of individual psychopathology. In the trainings for service providers done by GISST, the isolation brought on by social harassment and rejection is portrayed as a primary transgender health risk. This observation is supported by the interviews we conducted.

As do homosexual, lesbian, and bisexual youth, transgendered youth disproportionately end up on the streets or kill themselves, but they are invisible in statistics on youth homelessness and suicide (Garland and Zigler, 1993; Gibson, 1994 [1989]; Remafedi, Farrow, and Deisher, 1994 [1991]; Schneider, Farberow, and Kruks, 1994 [1989]). A transgendered activist noted that she had never met a transsexual or transgender who had not, at some time, talked about suicide. As several interviewees pointed out, engaging in risky behavior itself can be a slow form of suicide (see also Bockting, Rosser, and Coleman, 1993, p. 13, Bockting, Robinson, and Rosser 1998). Transgenders are ostracized by their families, in school, and on the streets. Many of those served by GISST dropped out of school to escape ridicule or as a consequence of fleeing home or being kicked out.

Among the majority of transgenders we interviewed, economic vulnerability due to lack of education is compounded by the difficulty of getting a job because of nonconforming gender appearance and of keeping a job during the slow transition to a more feminine self. Male-to-female transgenders frequently have trouble passing as women because changes undergone during the first puberty, such as the lowering of the voice and the growth of facial hair, do not reverse during the "second puberty" precipitated by hormones. According to transgenders we interviewed, the stress of trying to "pass" and avoid discovery or challenge is tremendous and contributes in significant ways to their inability to obtain or maintain legal employment.

As one obviously well-educated, middle-class transgender stated in a focus group,

> A normal woman, okay, she might worry about she's looking grim today. She's not worrying [someone interrupts: "About losing her job because of it!"]. . . She's not worrying about "Am I going to be read as a *woman* today!"

A transgender from a small New England town talked about how the stress of trying to pass and avoid detection drove her out of school:

> As time went on it got so frustrating having to wake up every morning like two hours early to pluck my facial hair and get ready. It was so time-consuming. Just a lot of pressure wondering, "Oh God, if I start to perspire a little bit are people going to see the shadow!" [Laughs nervously.] It's embarrassing. So just under the pressure I dropped out of school.

She continued by explaining how she then ended up in prostitution:

> So throughout that I needed means of money, and I had a couple of friends I met in this bar, and they were hustlers. They used to hustle in this park. They used to hustle there for money. I asked them if maybe they could introduce me to a couple of guys, you know, just a quick hand job for money. And I did it for a while.

> Then I decided to move to Boston because I used to travel back and forth with my transsexual friend, go to clubs. And I was propositioned down here, and it was a lot of money. I was offered a bill [$100], two bills. And it was worth it! I just went with it. It just became such easy money for doing so little.

So easy, and yet it is prostitution that leads many transgenders into alcohol and drug abuse.

For transgenders especially, participation in prostitution cannot be understood simply in economic terms. Hunger for identity affirmation is key to sex work as well as alcohol and drug abuse, as described by a focus group participant:

> See, when we all start in the beginning, it's not so much that we see it as prostitution. We see it as, for years, we've been ostracized for being little boys and being sissies. And then all of a sudden you walk into a place like [names two Boston bars that cater to transgenders], you put some makeup on, and you put a wig on, put some high heels on, and you're really startin' to let out what's inside. [Dramatic pause.] *And there's men there that want you!* I mean, it's more of an affirming thing, you know, maybe it's all lack of self-esteem or something. It gets into an ego trip. I mean, sooner or later it can kill you, or you get tired of it and you get out of it. But that's how it is in the beginning. It's "Wow, this man is fine, and he treated me like a girl!"

The risks of HIV transmission associated with the quest for a feminine body have already been discussed, and transgenders' sexual risk networks have also been introduced. What remains is to consider their dynamics of sexual encounters in more detail. First, it is important to note that sexual partners of transgenders served by GISST include commercial as well as noncommercial partners. Both private and paying sexual partners are part of transgenders' risk networks, yet some transgender sexual risks are without doubt heightened when sex is primarily for payment rather than pleasure. Safer-sex negotiation is short-circuited between transgenders and their sexual partners by numerous factors, which our respondents indicated are exacerbated in the context of prostitution.

Short-circuiting is manifested in two ways: either safer-sex negotiation is never initiated, which often happens, or, though initiated, it is not successful. For both transgenders and their sex partners, a negative self-image and associated alcohol and/or drug use can inhibit safer-sex negotiation. Moreover, clients can take advantage of transgendered sex workers' economic vulnerability and hunger for affirmation as women to obtain condomless sex, which many men consider to be more pleasurable.

A key risk-producing dynamic in encounters between transgenders and their sex partners is the meeting of conviction and confusion: many transgenders are convinced they are women, and many, if not most, know themselves to be heterosexual, whereas their partners are often conflicted about their sexual orientation and perhaps also their gender identity. Transgenders seek affirmation of their womanhood—their core personal identity—at the same time that their sex partners often seek a penis while denying that they are doing so. Transgenders may even risk HIV/AIDS for the sake of identity affirmation and to escape isolation through connection (see also Bockting, Rosser, and Coleman, 1993, p. 20).

For a transgender who has not had sex reassignment surgery, safer-sex negotiation might necessitate mention of her penis, which she may not want to mention because it conflicts with her female identity (see also Bockting, Rosser, and Coleman, 1993, p. 103). At the same time, if her sex partner wants her penis but cannot admit to himself that he does, he will not be able to openly discuss condom use. Thus, safer-sex negotiation is made more difficult by transgenders' female self-identity and by what one interviewee described as the "hidden homosexuality" of some of their sex partners. Risks are high: many transgenders are killed by clients or other sexual partners.[14] Safer-sex negotiations are complicated, whether inside or outside a commercial context, because the time that might be devoted to these negotiations is simply taken up by other issues, whether spoken or unspoken (see also Bockting, Rosser, and Coleman, 1993, p. 34). If, for example, a transgender is busy gauging how she is being read and what her sex partner might want but is unable to say, little room is left for safer-sex negotiation. When discrimination, economic vulnerability, and need for affirmation are taken into account, risk can be seen as affecting not a single individual but individuals in interaction, as arising from historical risk structures and perpetuated in contemporary risk networks.

This brings us to the fallacy of misplaced groupness, which can lead analysts to fail to distinguish between a category made by analysts and one formed by people themselves. Thus, a social category can be classified conceptually by analysts alone, for example, "poor women," or a social category can be classified conceptually by the members of that category themselves—transgender is only now emerging as an example of the latter. Only the latter involves identity. To understand why avoiding misplaced groupness is crucial to prevention, we need only recollect that when public health specialists mistook all men who engage in sex with men for a group called "homosexuals," prevention efforts failed to reach many behaviorally at risk.

TOWARD GROUP PREVENTION

The risk group model hinders *analysis* of how risk is shaped for individuals with complex identities who are situated in intricate developmental structures and interactional networks. Prevention *strategies,* on the other hand, are fostered by group identity and peer activism, as the example of the gay community in the United States has clearly shown. Thus, public health, whether anthropological or epidemiological, must shift analytical gears when moving from studying risk to promoting prevention. For prevention, identification with a group is beneficial, especially for the oppressed and/or minority groups so disproportionately affected by HIV/AIDS, other STIs, and substance abuse. Transgenders, the very example of the marginalized and despised, will be more healthy the more they identify as a group.

Our analysis of transgenders' historical and contemporary risk structures is an example of the move in social scientific study of health risks, especially for HIV infection, away from group and individual models toward understanding sociocultural determinants, a move echoing the best public health tradition begun in the last century. The recent anthropological volumes *Women, Poverty, and AIDS: Sex, Drugs, and Structural Violence* (Farmer, Connors, and Simmons, 1996) and *The Political Economy of AIDS* (Singer, 1998) are two examples among many. Such analyses point toward the root causes of ill health in cultural ideologies and institutions—in this case, our culture's dichotomous sex/gender system and derivative discrimination against those who transgress that system. They do not, however, suggest that all significant health interventions must address the pervasive and enduring social, economic, and political forces that create and perpetuate the inequalities on which health problems thrive. Although radical social change, as Jonathan Mann and others urge, is important, programs at other levels, especially programs that empower those at risk, are urgently needed. Such programs can help initiate precisely the large-scale sociocultural change that appears so intractable.

In June 1996, Rebecca Durkee organized the First New England Transgender Health Conference in Boston. Sponsored by the Massachusetts Department of Public Health, the conference was attended by over 200 service providers, educators, and transgenders from the New England region and beyond. Transgenders and others provided education and training on the health status of this critically underserved population. As transgenders recounted their journeys of survival and self-affirmation, other transgenders could see that their own problems were not the consequence of individual pathology, as psychologists would have it, but the patterned result of discrimination and rejection. And service providers and educators could understand how their own lack of knowledge and perhaps even prejudice contribute to the difficulties transgenders face.

The visibility and work of community-based advocates and organizations combat the isolation that transgenders feel. Both GISST and the Massachusetts-based International Foundation for Gender Education, an organization originally focused on male transvestites, receive frequent telephone calls from young people saying, "I thought I was the only one." Such individual interventions can be self-affirming and even lifesaving. In the closing session of the 1996 Transgender Health Conference, a transgender who performs in Boston's drag shows voiced a key theme of GISST's founder when she said that older transgenders must take care of younger ones to prevent them from suffering and even dying from the same risky behaviors she and others like her managed to survive.

Similar goals have been voiced by transgendered veterans of the streets elsewhere in the United States. For example, Kristine Withers (1995, p. 12), who does HIV/AIDS outreach in New York City and is active in "the transsexual civil rights struggle," reports:

> The very idea of getting off drugs and out of sex work was scary, but I couldn't do the streets any more. I had almost been killed seven times . . .

> In my vision, transsexuals [transgenders in the overarching terminology adopted here] would have something like the Lesbian and Gay Community Services Center. Gays and lesbians have come a long way. In terms of visibility, transsexuals are where Gays and Lesbians were twenty-five years ago, when transsexuals started it all [i.e., the Stonewall Rebellion, widely acknowledged in the gay, lesbian, and transgendered community as having been lead by transgenders (Feinberg, 1996, p. 9)].

> When I was coming up, I thought transsexuals could only do sex work because it was the only image I had seen. There was no other community for me as a transsexual and there were no professional transsexuals who were out or who I could look up to.

As I realized that there was a transsexual community, I saw that
I did have options and the street was no longer the only choice.

In June 1997, the Second New England Transgender Health Conference, also organized by Rebecca Durkee, was held in Boston. Attendance matched or surpassed that at the first conference. This turn-
out by providers and transgenders, including transgendered youth in
search of healthy identity affirmation, demonstrates the importance
of such educational and community-building events.

Rebecca Durkee's vision of a community of caring includes founding a transgender Alcoholics Anonymous group, promoting condom
distribution at the transgender bars, and running a series of trainings
on transgender health issues for providers throughout Massachusetts.
To eradicate the severe stigmatization that transgenders face from
childhood onward seems impossible, and yet the kinds of interventions and programs that Rebecca Durkee initiated through GISST
can contribute to that goal.

NOTES

1. Rebecca Durkee found a home for GISST at Beacon Hill Multicultural Association. Ms. Durkee currently consults on transgender and public health issues and
is writing a book on related topics.

2. HIV stands for human immunodeficiency virus, the infectious agent that precipitates the immune system breakdown that leads to a diagnosis of AIDS, acquired
immunodeficiency syndrome.

3. The 1997 advertisement compared Holiday Inn's recent renovations to a
transsexual's reconstructive surgery. In the 2000 advertisement for an e-business, a
drag queen pronounced a traditional business meeting a "drag."

4. It has been claimed that male-to-females vastly outnumbered female-to-
males (DSM-III-R cited in Denny, 1994, p. xxvi). In recent years, however, some
experts have suggested that "female to male gender dysphoria may be as common as
male to female" (Denny, 1994, p. xxviii; Griggs, 1998, p. 114), and there are some
reports that male-to-female and female-to-male surgeries are being done in about
equal numbers (Bornstein, 1994, p. 16). Since our interviewees included only one
female-to-male transsexual, we restrict our analysis to male-to-female transgenders.
Leslie Feinberg's (1993) fictional account in *Stone Butch Blues* suggests that, as
they grow up, female-to-male transgenders are subject to social stigmatization—
part of what we term here historical risk structures—similar to male-to-female
transgenders. We know that their social and sexual networks—what we label contemporary risk structures—differ. Female-to-male transgenders do not engage in
prostitution to the same extent as male-to-female transgenders both because there is
no ready clientele and because they can often pass more easily and can therefore get

legitimate employment. Their ability to pass more easily stems from the fact that the physical transformation with male hormones is more complete than with female hormones. With male hormones the voice lowers and body hair grows, whereas with female hormones the voice does not rise and the Adam's apple and facial hair do not disappear. As Claudine Griggs (1998, p. 81), a self-identified male-to-female transsexual, notes, the "bodies of female-to-male transsexuals are so effectively altered by hormone therapy that they are supremely confident in their attributions as men." This contrasts with many MTFs [male-to-females], who never escape the fear of being read [as a male]." For MTFs, secondary sexual characteristics that remain after hormone therapy can be altered: the voice by coaching and practice, the Adam's apple by a (surgical) tracheal shave, and the facial hair by an ordinary shave or electrolysis.

5. "Queen," in its most general usage, can refer to any male homosexual. When used by insiders, it need not carry a negative connotation, although it frequently does when used by outsiders. More narrowly, the term can be used for an effeminate homosexual male. Transsexuals and transgenders often refer to themselves as queens. "Drag queen," a synonym for female impersonator, applies to an anatomical male who wears female clothes in theatrical performance. Several of our interviewees stressed that in a drag show the drag queen lets it be known at some point that he is not really a woman, by dropping his voice down to its normal register or complaining about "tucking" (hiding his penis to prevent a bulge). One drag performer described this as a "wink" to the audience. The term "street queen" is usually used for a physiological man who lives as a woman and who has a street life, often involving prostitution and drug use. Street queens who are performers in drag shows are distinguished by Esther Newton (1972, p. 8) from drag queens by the fact that they "are never off stage"; that is, they always present as females on the stage and on the street. The rigidity of this distinction ignores the fact that financial, familial, and other constraints can prevent a street queen from presenting as female full-time.

6. Laws in the United States against female impersonation or cross-dressing have been stringent; people were arrested for wearing more than a specified number of articles of clothing of the opposite sex. Leslie Feinberg (1996, p.8), a biologically female transgender, reports:

> My greatest terror was always when the police raided the bars, because they had the law on their side. They *were* the law. It wasn't just the tie I was wearing or the suit that made me vulnerable to arrest. I broke the law every time I dressed in fly-front pants, or wore jockey shorts or t-shirts. The law dictated that I had to wear at least three pieces of "women's" clothing. My drag queen sisters had to wear three pieces of "men's" clothing. For all I know, that law may still be on the books in Buffalo today.

7. Many of the rest died of substance abuse-related problems (overdose or liver disease) or were murdered.

8. In using the words "prostitute" and "prostitution," whether applied to the United States or elsewhere, it is not our intention to stigmatize anyone. The trend in

epidemiological and scholarly literature is to use the terms "commercial sex worker" and "commercial sex work" instead (e.g., Celantano et al., 1993), with the thought apparently being that, unlike the terms "prostitute" and "prostitution," they are not stigmatizing. These labels are retained here to highlight the frequent harshness of work circumstances and coercion involved, whether individual (e.g., beatings, indenturing, kidnapping) or societal (e.g., stigma that contributes to prostitution among transgenders). To keep attention on the coercive rather than the capitalist dimensions of prostitution, we tend not to use the labels "commercial sex worker" and "commercial sex work."

9. Another form of self-medication that can involve the reuse of unsterilized needles is the injection of silicone or wax to augment the breasts (see also Bockting, Rosser, and Coleman, 1993, pp. 2, 34). We looked at electrolysis as a possible risk. If practiced according to professional standards, electrolysis needles are either dedicated to a particular person or disposable. Substandard practices, however, may pose a potential risk of HIV transmission.

10. As Packard and Epstein note (1992, p. 363), a study by Mann et al. (1986) found that seropositive children of seronegative mothers in Kinshasa, Zaire, had received more injections than their seronegative counterparts.

11. It is possible that, aside from the risks posed by hormone injections with re-used, unsterilized needles, these female hormones themselves may augment transgenders' susceptibility to HIV and other STIs. Medical experts believe that "hormonal changes during the menstrual cycle may make women more vulnerable to infection" (Berer, with Ray, 1993, p. 19).

12. See also articles in Aggleton's (1996) edited volume *Bisexualities and AIDS* for relevant case studies from Britain, Canada, India, and other countries.

13. Transvestism and transsexualism have been defined as medical and psychological conditions, with etiology sought in biology or family dynamics (Bolin, 1988; Denny, 1994, p. xxvii; Woodhouse, 1989). Explanations have been offered concerning hormonal deficiency, weak or absent fathers, and domineering mothers. But as Annie Woodhouse (1989, p. 75) observes in her ethnographic monograph on transvestites, "the seemingly endless search for causes may have little to offer." We would argue that focusing on etiology does not contribute to understanding transgenders' risks for alcohol and drug abuse and for HIV/AIDS and other STIs.

14. One such killing in the Boston area in 1995 was heralded with the headline "'Preppy' allegedly kills date in drag" and "Clean-cut computer worker charged in transsexual's killing" (*Boston Herald*, 1995, pp. 1, 12). Three of our interviewees have been killed since we completed our research.

REFERENCES

Aggleton, P., ed. *Bisexualities and AIDS: International Perspectives.* Bristol, PA: Taylor and Francis, 1996.

Alonso, A.M. and Koreck, M.T. Silences: "Hispanics," AIDS, and sexual practices. *Differences* 1(1):101-124, 1990.

American Psychiatric Association. *Diagnostic and Statistical Manual of Mental Disorders,* Third Edition. Washington, DC: American Psychiatric Association, 1980.

American Psychiatric Association. *Diagnostic and Statistical Manual of Mental Disorders,* Third Edition, Revised. Washington, DC: American Psychiatric Association, 1987.

American Psychiatric Association. *Diagnostic and Statistical Manual of Mental Disorders,* Fourth Edition. Washington, DC: American Psychiatric Association, 1994.

Berer, M. with Ray, S. *Women and HIV/AIDS: An International Resource Book.* London: Pandora Press, 1993.

Bockting, W., Robinson, B.E., and Rosser, B.R.S. Transgender HIV prevention: A qualitative needs assessment. *AIDS Care* 10(4):505-526, 1998.

Bockting, W., Rosser, B.R.S., and Coleman, E. *Transgender HIV/AIDS Prevention Program Manual.* Minneapolis: Program in Human Sexuality, Department of Family Practice and Community Health, Medical School, University of Minnesota, 1993.

Boles, J. and Elifson, K.W. The social organization of transvestite prostitution and AIDS. *Social Science and Medicine* 39(1):85-93, 1994.

Bolin, A. *In Search of Eve: Transsexual Rites of Passage.* South Hadley, MA: Bergin and Garvey Publishers, 1988.

Bolin, A. Transcending and transgendering: Male-to-female transsexuals, dichotomy, and diversity. In Herdt, G., ed., *Third Sex, Third Gender: Beyond Sexual Dimorphism in Culture and History.* New York: Zone Books, 1994, pp. 447-485.

Bornstein, K. *Gender Outlaw: On Men, Women, and the Rest of Us.* New York: Routledge, 1994.

Boston Herald. "Preppy" allegedly kills date in drag. *Boston Herald,* November 22, 1995, pp. 1, 12.

Boston Phoenix. Adult Services. *Boston Phoenix,* April 28, 1995, p. 13.

Carlson, R.G. and Siegal, H.A. The crack life: An ethnographic overview of crack use and sexual behavior among African-Americans in a midwest metropolitan city. *Journal of Psychoactive Drugs* 23(1):11-18, 1991.

Celantano, D.D., Nelson, K.E., Suprasert, S., Wright, N., Mantanasarawoot, A., Eiumtrakul, S., Romyen, S., Tulvatana, S., Kuntolbutra, S., Sirisopana, N. et. al. (1993). Behavioral and sociodemographic risks for frequent visits to commercial sex workers among northern Thai men. *AIDS,* 7(12), 1647-1652.

Connors, M. Risk perception, risk taking and risk management among intravenous drug users: Implications for AIDS prevention. *Social Science and Medicine* 34(6):591-601, 1992.

Denny, D. Gender dysphoria: A guide to research. *Garland Gay and Lesbian Studies,* Volume 10. New York: Garland Publishing, 1994.

Elifson, K.W., Boles, J., Posey, E., Sweat, M., Darrow, W., and Elsea, W. Male transvestite prostitutes and HIV Risk. *American Journal of Public Health* 83(2):260-262, 1993.

Errington, S. Recasting sex, gender, and power: A theoretical and regional overview. In Atkinson, J.M. and Errington, S., eds., *Power and Difference: Gender in Island Southeast Asia.* Stanford: Stanford University Press, 1990, pp. 1-58.

Farmer, P., Connors, M. and Simmons, J., eds. *Women, Poverty, and AIDS: Sex, Drugs, and Structural Violence.* Monroe, ME: Common Courage Press, 1996.

Fee, E. and Kreiger, N. Understanding AIDS: Historical interpretations and the limits of biomedical individualism. *American Journal of Public Health* 83(10): 1477-1486, 1993.

Feinberg, L. *Stone Butch Blues.* Ithaca, NY: Firebrand Books, 1993.

Feinberg, L. *Transgender Warriors: Making History from Joan of Arc to RuPaul.* Boston: Beacon Press, 1996.

Fry, P. Male homosexuality and spirit possession in Brazil. *Journal of Homosexuality* 11(3/4):137-153, 1985.

Garland, A. and Zigler, E. Adolescent suicide prevention: Current research and social policy implications. *American Psychologist* 48:169-182, 1993.

Gibson, P. Gay male and lesbian youth suicide. In Remafedi, G., ed., *Death by Denial: Studies of Suicide in Gay and Lesbian Teenagers.* Boston: Alyson Publications, 1994 [1989], pp. 15-68.

Griggs, C. *S/he: Changing Sex and Changing Clothes.* Oxford: Berg, 1998.

Herdt, G., ed. *Third Sex, Third Gender: Beyond Sexual Dimorphism in Culture and History.* New York: Zone Books, 1994.

Kane, S. and Mason, T. "IV drug users" and "sex partners": The limits of epidemiological categories and the ethnography of risk. In Herdt, E. and Lindenbaum, S., eds., *The Time of AIDS: Social Analysis, Theory, and Method.* Newbury Park, CA: Sage Publications, 1992, pp. 199-222.

Lancaster, R.N. "That we should all turn queer?" Homosexual stigma in the making of manhood and the breaking of a revolution in Nicaragua. In Parker, R.G. and Gagnon, J.H., eds., *Conceiving Sexuality: Approaches to Sex Research in a Postmodern World.* New York: Routledge, 1995, pp. 135-156.

Laumann, E.O. and Gagnon, J.H. A sociological perspective on sexual action. In Parker, R.G. and Gagnon, J.H., eds., *Conceiving Sexuality: Approaches to Sex Research in a Postmodern World.* New York: Routledge, 1995, pp. 183-213.

Lima, E.S., Friedman, S.R., Bastos, F.I., Telles, P.R., Friedmann, P., Ward, T.P., and DesJarlais, D.C. Risk factors for HIV-1 seroprevalence among drug injectors in the cocaine-using environment of Rio de Janeiro. *Addiction* 86(6): 689-698, 1994.

Mann, J.M. We are all Berliners: Notes from the Ninth International Conference on AIDS. *American Journal of Public Health* 83(10):1378-1379, 1993.

Mann, J.M. The future of the global AIDS movement. *Harvard AIDS Review* Spring:18-21, 1999.

Mann, J.M., Francis, H., Davachi, F., Baudoux, P., Quinn, T.C., Nzilambi, N., Bosenge, N., Colebunders, R.L., Piot, P., Kabote, N., et al. Risk factors for human immunodeficiency virus seropositivity among children 1-24 months old in Kinshasa, Zaire. *Lancet* 8508:654-657, 1986.

Mason, T.H., Connors, M.M., and Kammerer, C.A. *Transgenders and HIV Risks: Needs Assessment.* Boston: Gender Identity Support Services for Transgenders, prepared for the Massachusetts Department of Public Health, HIV/AIDS Bureau, 1995.

Morris, M., Podhisita, C., Wawer, M.J., and Handcock, M.S. Bridge populations in the spread of HIV/AIDS in Thailand. *AIDS* 10(11):1265-1271, 1996.

Morse, E.V., Simon, P.M, Osofsky, H.J., Balson, P.M., and Gaumer, H.R. The male street prostitute: A vector for transmission of HIV infection into the heterosexual world. *Social Science and Medicine* 32(5):535-539, 1991.

Nangeroni, N.R. *Transgenderism.* Cambridge, MA. Ninja Design, 1995 <nrn@world.std.com>.

Newton, E. *Mother Camp: Female Impersonation in America.* Englewood Cliffs, NJ: Prentice-Hall, 1972.

Oppenheimer, G.M. In the eye of the storm: The epidemiological construction of AIDS. In Fee, E. and Fox, D.M., eds., *AIDS: The Burdens of History.* Berkeley: University of California Press, 1988, pp. 267-300.

Oppenheimer, G.M. Causes, cases, and cohorts: The role of epidemiology in the historical construction of AIDS. In Fee, E. and Fox, D.M., eds., *AIDS: The Making of a Chronic Disease.* Berkeley: University of California Press, 1992, pp. 49-83.

Packard, R.M. and Epstein, P. Medical research on AIDS in Africa: A historical perspective. In Fee, E. and Fox, D.M., eds., *AIDS: The Making of a Chronic Disease.* Berkeley: University of California Press, 1992, pp. 346-376.

Panos Institute. *The Third Epidemic: Repercussions of the Fear of AIDS.* London: Panos Institute, in association with the Norwegian Red Cross, 1990.

Parker, R.G. Masculinity, femininity, and homosexuality: On the anthropological interpretation of sexual meanings in Brazil. *Journal of Homosexuality* 11(3/4): 155-163, 1985.

Parker, R.G. Youth, identity, and homosexuality: The changing shape of sexual life in contemporary Brazil. *Journal of Homosexuality* 17(3/4):268-289, 1989.

Parker, R.G. *Bodies, Pleasures, and Passions: Sexual Culture in Contemporary Brazil.* Boston: Beacon Press, 1991.

Raymond, J. *The Transsexual Empire: The Making of the She-Male.* New York: Teachers College Press, 1994 [1979].

Remafedi, G., Farrow, J.A., and Deisher, R.W. Risk factors for attempted suicide in gay and bisexual youth. In Remafedi, G., ed., *Death by Denial: Studies of Suicide in Gay and Lesbian Teenagers.* Boston: Alyson Publications, 1994 [1991], pp. 123-137.

Rothblatt, M. *The Apartheid of Sex: A Manifesto on the Freedom of Gender.* New York: Crown Publishers, 1995.

Rothenberg, R. and Narramore, J. The relevance of social network concepts to sexually transmitted disease control. *Sexually Transmitted Diseases* 23(1):24-29, 1996.

Sankary, T.M., Ichikawa, S., Kondo, M., Imai, M., Ohya, H., Kihara, M., and Kihara, M. Sentinel surveillance of HIV molecular clones in condom semen samples from clients of female prostitutes in Japan. *International Conference on AIDS* 11(1):145 (abstract no. Mo.C.1520), 1996, July 7-12.

Schiller, N.G. What's wrong with this picture? The hegemonic construction of culture in AIDS research in the United States. *Medical Anthropology Quarterly* 6(3):237-254, 1992.

Schiller, N.G., Crystal, S., and Dewellen, D. Risky business: The cultural construction of AIDS risk groups. *Social Science and Medicine* 38(10):1337-1346, 1994.

Schneider, S.G., Farberow, N.L., and Kruks, G.N. Suicidal behavior in adolescent and young adult gay men. In Remafedi, G., ed., *Death by Denial: Studies of Suicide in Gay and Lesbian Teenagers*. Boston: Alyson Publications, 1994 [1989], pp. 107-122.

Singer, M., ed. *The Political Economy of AIDS*. Amityville, NY: Baywood Publishing, 1998.

Strunin, L. and Hingson, R. Alcohol, drugs, and adolescent sexual behavior. *International Journal of the Addictions* 27(2):126-146, 1992.

Stuart, K.E. *The Uninvited Dilemma: A Question of Gender*. Portland, OR Metamorphous Press, 1991.

Treichler, P.A. AIDS, homophobia, and biomedical discourse: An epidemic of significance. In Crimp, D., ed., *AIDS: Cultural Analysis/Cultural Activism*. Cambridge: MIT Press, 1988 [1987], pp. 33-70.

Weeks, J. History, desire, and identities. In Parker, R.G. and Gagnon, J.H., eds., *Conceiving Sexuality: Approaches to Sex Research in a Postmodern World*. New York: Routledge, 1995, pp. 33-50.

Withers, K. Notes from a survivor. *LAP Notes* (Lesbian AIDS Project, Gay Men's Health Crisis) 3:12, 1995.

Wood, M.M., Rhodes, F., and Malotte, C.K. Pilot study of drug-using men who have sex with men: Access and intervention strategies. *International Conference on AIDS* 11(1):337 (abstract no. Tu.C.2412), July 7-12, 1996.

Woodhouse, A. *Fantastic Women: Sex, Gender, and Transvestism*. New Brunswick, NJ: Rutgers University Press, 1989.

Chapter 3

Transgender Health and Social Service Needs in the Context of HIV Risk

Nina Kammerer
Theresa Mason
Margaret Connors
Rebecca Durkee

INTRODUCTION

This chapter draws on an HIV/AIDS needs assessment of the transgender community of Boston conducted by three of the authors and on the experiences of the fourth author. In 1995, Theresa Mason, Margaret Connors, and Nina Kammerer, all medical anthropologists who have done AIDS research in the United States or abroad, were commissioned to do the needs assessment by Rebecca Durkee, founder of Gender Identity Sup-

We are all grateful to the Massachusetts Department of Public Health AIDS Bureau for funding the needs assessment of Boston's transgender community. We are deeply indebted to every individual who was interviewed or participated in a focus group. This chapter is a revision and expansion of sections of *Transgenders and HIV Risk: Needs Assessment* (Mason, Connors, and Kammerer, 1995). An earlier version was presented at the 1997 American Anthropological Association Annual Meeting, Washington, DC, as part of the panel "Transgender Identity, Community Building, and Health." Our thanks to members of the audience, in particular David Valentine, for their helpful comments. This chapter was originally published on the Internet in the *International Journal of Transgenderism,* 3(1), January-March 1999 <http://www.symposion. com/ijt/hiv-risk/kammerer. html>. We are grateful to Drs. Walter Bockting and Sheila Kirk, the editors of that special issue, for their comments on a draft. We are also grateful to Dr. Bockting for arranging hard-copy publication.

Correspondence and requests for materials should be addressed to Nina Kammerer at <nkammerer@har.org>.

port Services for Transgenders (GISST), an advocacy and service program located in Boston.[1] The Massachusetts Department of Public Health, HIV/AIDS Bureau funded the study. Our research and the resultant report focused on the segment of the transgender community served by GISST, namely, economically and psychologically vulnerable male-to-female transsexual and transgendered individuals, many of whom end up on the street at some point in their lives, engaging in commercial and survival sex (Mason, Connors, and Kammerer, 1995).

Central to our research was unraveling the structuring of risk for HIV infection among transgenders. Transgenders' sexual and injection risks for HIV arise from three main sources: (1) social stigma and related negative self-image, (2) economic vulnerability and related prostitution and substance abuse, and (3) the quest for a feminine body and the need for identity affirmation. We found that for many economically vulnerable male-to-female transgenders, substance abuse was precipitated by participation in prostitution, rather than the other way around. Transgenders' needle risks for HIV stem not only from the injection of illicit drugs but also from the injection of hormones for bodily transformation or of silicone for breast augmentation as part of the quest for a feminine body. The need for identity affirmation through sexual expression can lead to unsafe sex.

Elsewhere we discuss transgenders' HIV risks (Mason, Connors, and Kammerer, 1995; Kammerer et al., in Chapter 2 of this book). The focus here is on the kinds of health and social services transgenders require, problems specific to the transgender community in obtaining such services, and, finally, insights that providers and transgenders themselves have into how services can be improved, especially in AIDS prevention and risk reduction.

In this chapter, the noun "transgender" and the adjective "transgendered" are used broadly, encompassing individuals who self-identify as transsexual, whether preoperative, postoperative, or nonoperative, that is, not desirous of having sex reassignment surgery, and individuals who self-identify as transgender. Our research focused not on transvestites who cross-dress but on transgenders who cross-live (Woodhouse, 1989). Since the 1980s, a grassroots political movement, sometimes labeled transgenderism (Rothblatt, 1995, p. 16), has grown up seeking transgender rights and affirming transgender pride (Bolin, 1994; Feinberg, 1996). For many in the transgender—or "trans"—movement, the label transgender encompasses not only transsexuals and transgenders, as it does here, but also cross-dressers or transvestites, drag queens, intersexed individuals, and anyone nonconventionally gendered (Feinberg, 1996). For some, trans unity is within the "queer" nation, with the term queer being expanded from meaning homosexual only to meaning nonconventional sexual orientation and/or gender identity (Valentine, forthcoming).

After describing our anthropological research methods, we consider health and social service needs. Our contention is that the difficulties transgenders have in gaining access to shelters, securing safety in prisons, and obtaining appropriate mental health counseling, as well as other health and social services, are related to their risk of HIV infection. This is a continuation of our argument, outlined earlier, that discrimination and social stigma shape transgenders' HIV risk behaviors. Next we identify and correct some misinterpretations held by health and social service providers that contribute to transgenders' difficulties in obtaining caring and appropriate services. We conclude with specific recommendations for HIV prevention and risk reduction, particularly for the most economically vulnerable male- to-female transgenders, who often end up on the streets and/or in prostitution. HIV prevention by and for transgenders can help reduce the incidence of AIDS at the same time that it provides positive role models and contributes to community building.

RESEARCH METHODS

Adhering to an ethnographic research approach, we attempted to understand HIV risks and health and social service needs from transgenders' and service providers' perspectives. Between April and August 1995, the researchers conducted focus groups and open-ended interviews with transgenders and interviews with health and social service providers. In addition, we visited three transgender bar scenes in person to observe firsthand. One of us also attended two trainings for providers, led by Rebecca Durkee, on transgender health issues in a statewide series funded by the Massachusetts Department of Public Health.

Transgendered interviewees and focus group participants ranged in age from late teens to sixties. They included African Americans and Anglo Americans, as well as a Latina living with AIDS, an eighteen-year-old recently arrived in Boston and currently a street sex worker, an Anglo former escort service sex worker, and four local ac-

tivists. We interviewed one female-to-male, in part to clarify the variet-
ies of transgenderism. The service providers interviewed all worked in
the field of HIV prevention and/or services for street youth.

Although the data focus on the economically most vulnerable
transgenders, some of the findings, especially concerning the barriers
that stigma and discrimination pose to appropriate care (Green,
Brinken, and HRC Staff, 1994), are likely to be valid even for more
economically advantaged transgenders. Similarly, while the findings
cannot be assumed to be applicable to female-to-male transgenders,
other sources suggest that discrimination diminishes the quantity and
quality of care they receive.[2]

HEALTH AND SOCIAL SERVICE NEEDS

Transgenders, whom one activist called "the orphans of the orphans," have great difficulty with access to health and social services.
Even when transgenders do gain access, their difficulties continue,
since providers frequently do not understand them and their needs.
Aside from GISST, Enterprise (for female-to-male transsexuals), and
Boston Alliance of Gay, Lesbian, Bisexual, and Transgender Youth
(BAGLY), only one Boston service provider, the Fenway Community Health Center's Color Me Healthy program, explicitly targeted
transgenders at the time of our research.

The economically vulnerable male-to-female transgenders who
were the focus of our needs assessment reported that they rarely seek
medical care, except as it relates to their quest for a feminine body.
There are numerous reasons for this, with lack of insurance and lack
of acceptance prominent among them. Transgenders' fears of rejection by medical practitioners and facilities are founded either on personal experience or on gossip about the degrading and even dangerous
encounters that others similar to themselves have had with doctors
and hospitals. One self-identified preoperative transsexual told a hor-
rifying story of being sent away from a well-known Boston emergency room after a car accident, even though she was suffering from
serious injuries, including fractured vertebrae and a concussion.
When her male genitalia were discovered under her female clothing,
she was discharged without treatment!

Transgenders know well from experience or from their peers that
"homeless shelters won't let a queen in. They say 'dress like a man or

get the hell out!' So you're forced back into the element," that is, back onto the street. Staff at shelters will not accept male-to-female transgenders in women's shelters, and most will not permit them in men's shelters unless they wear men's clothes. If transgenders are allowed to wear their own clothes in men's shelters, they are subject to derision and possible violence by fellow clients and sometimes by staff. Even if they disguise their core personal identities by dressing in men's clothes, they still run these risks. Service providers interviewed attested that it was nearly impossible to refer transgenders to shelters; one even used the adjective "ludicrous." This same provider reported that when he worked in Worcester, the state's second largest city, he could not find shelters willing to take transgenders but could sometimes find sympathetic service providers willing to put them up in their own homes for a night. Rosie's Place, a shelter for women in Boston, has accepted at least one male-to-female transgender.

Boston has no alcohol or drug treatment groups or facilities specifically for transgenders. Some find support in twelve-step programs run for and by the gay community; yet historical friction between transgenders and the gay community means that this is not always a workable fit.[3] Residential detoxification programs present the same problems as homeless shelters: transgenders are rarely placed in women's programs, and in men's programs they are either forced to hide their core personal identities or risk scorn and possible physical abuse. The only case we learned about of a male-to-female transgender being placed in a women's program was for Worcester, rather than Boston. As one interviewee said, "[We] can't get into detox without going completely against our nature. How would you like to be called 'sir' all day long?"

Obviously, the problems for transgenders in prison are similar and likely to be more serious. Only those few who have completed sex reassignment surgery *and* legally changed their sex from male to female on their birth certificates, which is, in fact, only possible in some states, would be put in a women's prison (Stuart, 1991, pp. 67, 71). In a men's correctional institution, male-to-female transgenders are vulnerable to various forms of abuse, including forced sex with inmates or guards. One of the respondents in a focus group who had recently gotten out of prison told such stories, observing that when she complained to a guard she was told to "deal," since the guard felt that she was the one who wanted to be a woman. The risk of physical abuse, including sexual abuse, is very real, not only inside correctional institutions, but outside in society. Some interviewees told of being forced to have sex with prison guards or others whose duty was supposed to be to protect them, while others told of being physically assaulted on the street. Lacking financial resources and knowing society's disdain for them, these individuals do not seek redress through the legal system.

According to service providers, transgenders are disproportionately represented among street youth, as are gays and lesbians. Given that problems in school and at home often contribute to a young person being on the street, this disproportionate representation is not surprising. Unfortunately, however, we found only one self-identified transgender service provider working directly with youth in the Boston metropolitan area. Fortunately, however, Boston's providers of services to street youth recognize the need for transgendered workers, although they have had difficulty finding and retaining such workers.

To get off the streets, transgenders, whether youth or adults, need jobs to provide the financial resources to pay for housing, food, and other necessities. Society, however, makes it extremely difficult for transgenders to hold down jobs, especially those who do not "pass" well. Job training and placement are thus useless unless accompanied by efforts to ensure that transgenders will be retained on the job even with a five-o'clock shadow. Such efforts would need to include education to alter social attitudes toward transgenders and legal changes to prevent and punish discrimination against them. Currently, such discrimination is not illegal. Transgenders often have trouble getting on welfare because, as one provider explained, "from the minute you write in your name, welfare will say, 'No, what's your real name?' And right there it's downhill."

The social stigma that transgenders face from early in life is translated via internalization and fear into psychological problems, notably, low self-esteem and even loathing, often to the point of suicidal tendencies. Transgenders are thus frequently in need of sensitive and knowledgeable counseling. Unfortunately, their issues and problems are often little understood by providers of psychological services. One service provider, who had himself sought such services in his youth, noted that in practice,

> [s]ervice providers who serve adolescents really don't encourage people to experiment far from the norm. . . . I think they say, "Well, this is nice and everything, *but* your goal is to act as con-

ventional as possible by the time you're out of our hands." . . .
So it's like, "That sounds great and everything, but ditch the eye
makeup," you know?

Although this comment was made with respect to providers of services to adolescents, similar failures to acknowledge and respect the
seriousness of transgender issues can also be found among counselors serving adult transgenders.

Various forms of outreach that might be thought to serve transgenders do not do so effectively. For example, given the existence of
friction between the gay and transgender communities and the fact
that most transgenders do not self-identify as gay, gay organizations
can have trouble reaching them. It is also important to point out, as
one gay service provider did, that gays are not necessarily any more
knowledgeable about transgenders and their issues than anyone else.
After listening to a colleague give a nuanced and thorough overview
of transsexual, transgender, and related categories, he commented, "I
can tell you that the average gay man living in the South End [a neighborhood in Boston] would not have said anything other than people
who have a sex change operation." His colleague, himself a drag performer, pointed out that gay men also mistake transgenders for drag
queens, that is, for homosexual men who wear women's clothes for
performance (see Newton, 1972).

Organizations that target prostitutes often are run by women for
women, and transgenders are left out. As Janice Raymond's attack on
transsexuals in her book *The Transsexual Empire* testifies, some
women, more particularly, some feminists and lesbian feminists, are
antagonistic toward transsexuals—"artificial women" in Raymond's
(1994 [1979], p. 69) terms—because they are seen as representing a
retrogressive vision of womanhood.

Cruising zones for female, gay, and transgendered commercial sex
workers are geographically separate. One particular Boston neighborhood is known as the transgender zone; indeed, one transgendered interviewee said that she assumes that any man who does a pickup there
knows that the prostitute is transgendered. This geographical specializa-
tion means that outreach workers in a zone traditionally used by women
sex workers or by gay street hustlers are not likely to encounter
transgendered sex workers. The same is true for drug outreach. Although many transgenders have drug problems, they are not reached by

services targeted to the drug-using population because, as one transgender observed, "they are in different areas, keep different hours."

Another reason that transgenders may not be reached effectively
by drug outreach is that, in the words of one service provider, it is for
"people who are about needles" and transgenders are not primarily
about needles. Thus, transgenders often "don't identify as drug users
. . . even though they're using a pretty high amount of recreational
drugs." Their primary issue is a "gender issue," rather than drug use.
People who are about needles are likely to go to substance abuse outreach workers who "talk that talk." What transgenders need is outreach workers who talk gender issue talk.

Despite the significant HIV/AIDS risks faced by transgenders, we
could locate targeted prevention programs in only a handful of locations throughout the country. Besides Ms. Durkee's work locally in
Boston and statewide in Massachusetts, these programs include efforts
in Minneapolis, Minnesota (Bockting, Rosser, and Coleman, 1993);
San Francisco, California (Green, Brinken, and HRC Staffs, 1994,
p. 29; Lockett, 1995, p. 213); New York City (Withers, 1995; PWAC of
New York, 1996, p. 38); and Philadelphia, Pennsylvania, where
ActionAIDS (1994) has Care in Action Transgendered Program,
which includes street outreach, a telephone information line, and support groups by transgenders for transgenders. In Boston, no AIDS
prevention messages are posted at the primary drag queen and
transgender bar. Transgenders report that condoms distributed free to
this establishment are kept out of sight behind the bar, instead of being openly available on the counter, as in many other bars. As of
1995, GISST was the only transgender organization locally, or, indeed, in Massachusetts as a whole, dedicated to HIV/AIDS prevention for this community.

Once transgenders are infected with HIV, they confront the problem with which this section began, namely, lack of access to standard
medical care. One HIV-positive self-identified transsexual interviewee,
who is unusual in having the benefit of membership in a health main-
tenance organization (HMO), recounted a sad saga of trying to find a
participating physician to treat her. She called every provider listed in
a lengthy booklet sent out by her HMO. Some hung up on her; others
refused to accept her as a patient. She found only one doctor on the
list willing to take her on as a patient. Fortunately for her, he was not
only willing to treat her but was also familiar with transsexuality,

having worked in the past at The Johns Hopkins Gender Identity Clinic. What would she have done if she hadn't found him?

PROBLEMS IN OBTAINING APPROPRIATE SERVICES

Problems in obtaining services, such as discrimination, lack of acceptance, and absence of legal protection, are already evident from the preceding discussion. Many of these stem from the social stigma carried by transgenders. For example, placement in shelters for either women or men would not be a problem if society accepted transgenders wholeheartedly. Here we correct some misperceptions commonly held by service providers that may inhibit the provision of appropriate health and social services. Before so doing, we want to stress that in our interviews with Boston area providers we found great concern about transgender issues, overwhelming interest in learning more about transgenders and their needs, and sincere desire to improve and expand services for them. In this spirit, we identify some misperceptions that can hamper the efforts of well-intentioned providers.

To Be Transgendered Is Not Necessarily to Be Gay

Transgenderism concerns gender identity rather than sexual orientation (Bolin, 1988, p. 13; Stuart, 1991, p. 5; Griggs, 1998, p. 1). There are heterosexual, bisexual, and homosexual transgenders, though sources report that the majority of transgenders are heterosexual (Stuart, 1991, p. 55). Some providers equate transgendered gender identity with gay sexual orientation. Yet information and approaches appropriate to gay men may not fit the many transgenders who are not homosexual and may be ignored or actively rejected by them.

Historically, transgenders have gravitated to gay spaces and communities, where, as Stuart (1991, p. 41) observes, they "find some measure of acceptance." Indeed, some transgenders not only spend time within the gay community but also consider themselves gay for at least a period of their lives. Stuart (1991, p. 47) reports that most of the heterosexually identified transsexuals she interviewed "had explored the homosexual world." Some male-to-female transgenders consider themselves gay men, only later to realize and/or acknowledge that they are female rather than effeminate. As the category transgender becomes more widely known, this phenomenon of a gay phase in the life cycle of those transgenders whose sexual orientation is not homosexual may become less common.

Given the coexistence of transgenders and gays in the same social space and the gay phase in some transgenders' lives, it is easy for service providers and others to mistakenly equate being transgendered with being gay. It is also important to point out that what appears to outsiders as a same-sex encounter may be perceived by one or more of the partners as heterosexual. Thus, for a heterosexually self-identified male-to-female transgender, whether possessing male genitalia or surgically constructed female genitalia, having sexual intercourse with a genetic male is a heterosexual act: she is a woman having sex with a man.

Many, Perhaps Most, Transgenders Do Not Consider Themselves Drag Queens

Another misreading found among the gay community and elsewhere is to equate transgenders with drag queens. Drag queens, as one gay service provider who is himself a drag performer explained, "do it for the show only—they don't try to pass in real life—and the whole purpose of the show is look . . . there's a wink that goes on with the audience through the whole show." Even those male-to-female transgenders for whom life's exigencies—"grave concern over the potential loss of jobs, family, and friends" (Griggs, 1998, p. 39)—prohibit living full-time as women are not dressing for show but, rather, to express their core gender identities. To read a transgender as a drag queen is to trivialize her female self-identity, misinterpreting it as simply dress or performance.

In sum, a drag queen, in the sense of a cross-dressing performer, may identify as a woman while dressed as one. However, transgenders, by definition, experience their gender as either distinct from or in opposition to their biological sex all the time. This is true even if they are unable to live out that gender identity full-time. Some transgenders do perform in drag shows. Since transgendered performers and gay drag queens often share the same stage, equating the two is an easy mistake for outsiders to make. Some transgenders self-identify as drag queens, while recognizing their difference from their fellow drag queens who are nontransgendered. Some transgenders and gay drag queens insist on remaining united within the trans movement. At the Stonewall 25 march, in which drag queens were placed in front and transgenders further back, one transgender carried a sign reading "**DRAG** AND **TRANSGENDER** WILL **NOT** BE DIVIDED. QUEER **UNITY** = HUMAN **RIGHTS**" (Feinberg, 1996, p. 99, photo and caption, emphasis in the original).

Male-to-Female Transgenders Do Not Necessarily Live Full-Time As Women

At least one service provider defined transsexuals as living as the opposite gender full-time. It is important to remember that many exigencies, financial and otherwise, can prevent a male-to-female transgender from always dressing as a woman, even if she wants to. So it would be wrong to assume that a genetically male individual presenting at a service provider in men's clothes could not be a male-to-female transgender.

Transgendered interviewees reported that some providers believe that some or all transgendered prostitutes wear women's clothes to attract clients and/or get more money per trick. This view depicts female presentation of self as something put on and thereby refuses to recognize that, for transgenders, wearing women's clothes is an expression of their core personal identities. It is possible that this view derives either from the misinterpretation of transgenders as gay or as drag queens or from a mistaken analogy between them and those male street hustlers whose sexual orientation is heterosexual but who act homosexual for money, engaging in sex with men only when hustling.

Transgenders' Adolescent Confusion Is Not the Same As Other Adolescents' Confusion

An additional misperception is to equate transgenders' adolescent problems with typical adolescent soul-searching and rebelliousness. On the surface, the confusion of a nontransgendered adolescent who is experimenting with identities and/or sexual orientations may appear similar to that of a transgendered adolescent. Yet they spring from vastly different sources, and transgenders can suffer from both sorts of confusion.

Adolescence is recognized as a time of searching, experimentation, and rebellion, as self-identity is defined and independence established. An adolescent, whether transgendered or not, may be unsure of his or her identity. Yet a significant difference exists between confusion arising from not knowing who you are and confusion arising from a disjuncture between your personal self-knowledge and the categories and roles society presents and accepts. Whereas the confusion of a typical teenager falls into the first, the so-called confusion specific to a transgendered teenager falls into the second.

Transgenders typically know themselves to be different from an early age (Stuart, 1991, pp. 38-50), as young as three years old for one of our informants. As Griggs (1998, p. x), herself a male-to-female transsexual, notes, most of her transsexual informants "believe that it is something they were born with." Transgenders may not have the categories with which to think about and understand their difference until much later in life, however. For such individuals, knowing that there are others similar to themselves can be a lifeline that, quite literally, prevents them from committing suicide. Vivian Allen, formerly of the Waltham-based International Foundation for Gender Education (IFGE), reported that "every day someone calls up and says, 'Oh, my God, I thought I was the only one.' "

During one of the 1995 state-funded trainings on transgender health, Grace Sterling Stowell of the Boston Alliance of Gay, Lesbian, Bisexual, and Transgender Youth emphasized the difference between playing with gender identity and/or sexual orientation as part of adolescent exploration and "seriously exploring" sexual orientation by gay, lesbian, and bisexual youth and gender identity by transgendered youth. What it means to provide a safe space for playful adolescent exploration and for serious exploration is different. Many service providers steer clear of labels—gay, lesbian, heterosexual, homosexual, and the like—so that adolescents can find themselves, rather than being pigeonholed by others.[4] Yet categories may be precisely what youthful transgenders need to help them name what they already know but for which they have no label. For transgendered youth to discover other transgenders can be transformative, as one transsexual we interviewed recounted:

> And then I had met a transsexual. . . . I met her and I saw a little of myself in her. I looked at her, admired her for her going out and doing what she wanted to do for her self-comfortability [sic], and how she saw herself within.

Shifting identities, often including a period of gay self-identification, are evident in the life histories of transgenders obtained by us and by other researchers (e.g., Stuart, 1991, pp. 47-48). These must be understood, at least in part, as expressions, not of fluid personal identity, but of the quest for a fit between individual self-perception and social categories. There are no commonly accepted social categories for who transgenders are. Transgendered adolescents confused about where they fit into society may well need affirmation that they are not experimenting but, rather, are expressing their fundamental personal identities. This affirmation may be particularly important coming from service providers. It may help transgenders to avoid seeking social acceptance in risky ways, including through unprotected sexual encounters with male paying or nonpaying partners who treat them like women (Mason, Connors, and Kammerer, 1995; Kammerer et al., this book).

Male-to-Female Transgenders Are Not Necessarily Feminists

Providers can go overboard in affirming the womanhood of a male-to-female transgender. That a transgender considers herself a woman does not mean that she is a feminist. A feminist and/or lesbian may not be the most appropriate service provider for "a queen," who, in the words of one interviewee, " tries to be the perfect girl," whose idea of femininity may be retrogressive from a feminist and/or lesbian perspective. At one of the 1995 trainings on transgender health issues, a service provider recognized that assigning a male-to-female transsexual to a radical lesbian service provider was a mismatch.

IMPLICATIONS AND RECOMMENDATIONS FOR HIV PREVENTION

Both transgenders and service providers pointed to community building as the foundation not only for HIV/AIDS prevention but also for improved health and social services in general for transgenders. Pointing to the model of the gay community, they stressed that without a strong sense of community and mutual responsibility transgenders cannot get the kind of support they need as individuals. In addition, they pointed out that self-respect and pride promote changes in social attitudes toward members of the community by outsiders, which, in turn, foster self-respect. Since many HIV/AIDS risks among transgenders arise from social stigma and resultant self-loathing, community building is fundamentally related to HIV/

AIDS prevention, as well as to other health and social service needs (Mason, Connors, and Kammerer, 1995; Kammerer et al., this book). Transgenders and providers also identified having transgendered leaders and role models, transgendered outreach workers, transgender twelve-step programs, transgender support groups, and trainings in transgender health such as those conducted in Massachusetts in 1995 as being vital to HIV/AIDS prevention and to improving health and social services more broadly.

The following recommendations draw on the needs assessment and Rebecca Durkee's community-based work in HIV/AIDS prevention.

Training on Transgender Issues

To create a more socially accepting and supportive environment for transgenders most at risk of HIV infection, key HIV-related service providers should be trained in, and sensitized to, transgender perspectives, issues, and circumstances. A curriculum on HIV prevention for transgenders was developed from the 1995 state-funded provider trainings in Massachusetts (Durkee, 1995). The trainings themselves, which were well attended and highly rated by service providers, involved transgendered volunteers, including one woman living with AIDS. These volunteers spoke in public, in some cases for the first time, about the tremendous challenges they have faced with different facets of the health and social service systems. Such trainings clearly need to be continued in Massachusetts and inaugurated elsewhere. Given staff turnover at health and social service providers, they should be offered on a regular basis.

Transgender-Targeted HIV Prevention Outreach

Outreach is needed to the streets and bars where transgenders commonly encounter "tricks" or sexual partners. The outreach should be conducted by transgender-identified individuals themselves to establish the connections of trust and rapport necessary for the HIV education and risk reduction process to have an impact. This is also imperative because of transgenders' tremendous need for role models and for developing a sense of community. Transgenders offering escort service advertisements in local papers, such as the *Boston Phoenix,* should also be targeted. Outreach is a crucial aspect of HIV prevention among those who have been marginalized and who must struggle with poor self-images. The outreach teams should be ethnically mixed to facilitate engaging the diversity of transgenders in a variety of neighborhoods, especially the younger and perhaps more isolated ones. Collaborations should be pursued with local agencies that may be intersecting with, but perhaps not adequately addressing, transgenders in their areas. In the Boston metropolitan area, for example, an agency such as Centro Hispano de Chelsea, which is already involved with Latino cross-dressers, might be enlisted.

Risk Network-Targeted HIV Prevention

Outreach should also work to have an impact on the customers at the bars and the clients of transgender prostitutes as well. An advantage of having transgendered outreach workers in the prostitute stroll areas is the likelihood that they would be approached by clients and could begin the process of making them more aware of the need for prevention, providing them with condoms and HIV educational brochures. A transgender outreach worker should visit the transgender bars on weekend evenings and on special event nights, which draw a larger clientele. These outreach workers would carry around baskets of condoms and generally strive to integrate the spirit, vocabulary, and materials of HIV prevention into these scenes. Another suggestion is to introduce educational skits containing HIV prevention messages into the shows by transgendered and drag performers. This would have a powerful impact on the culture of the bars. The need to engage the bars in the HIV education and risk reduction process can be advanced by recruiting bar managers onto the boards of transgender community-based organizations, as was done in Boston.

Transgender-Appropriate HIV Prevention Literature

Another clear need is for the development of HIV prevention materials, such as posters, brochures, and risk reduction packets, targeted to transgenders. The tone and imagery, as well as the information, should take into account the serious need for transgenders to feel that they matter, that their health and safety are important, and that they have the power to protect themselves. Such materials should be posted and available in bars and clubs, and in health and social service agencies utilized by transgenders. Risk reduction packets could also be created to be handed out to the street sex workers and those transgenders frequenting bars.

Social Acceptance and Support

Outreach is also needed as a means of engaging transgenders, especially transgendered youth, in a process of self-assessment and psychological support. Drawing individuals into an office or a space where they can feel comfortable or offering parties during which HIV education messages are conveyed can also encourage the empowering experience of feeling noticed and taken seriously. All of this can further advance the goals of HIV prevention.

These five recommendations are made in recognition of the substantial HIV risks faced by transgenders, especially male-to-female transgenders involved in prostitution and related substance abuse. The current near-absence of HIV/AIDS prevention for transgenders in Boston and throughout the United States can be attributed in part to the invisibility of this population and to its social and economic marginalization. Due to that marginalization, it does not have the wherewithal to protect itself without outside assistance. Interviews with activists belonging to the economically more secure segment of the transgender community revealed an unwillingness to confront HIV/AIDS head-on, despite a recognition that male cross-dressers— transvestites—and economically well-off transgenders face risks similar to risks faced by their less affluent transgendered sisters. As Vivian Allen, previously of the International Foundation for Gender Education, put it, "the problem always is ownership." More affluent transgenders are loath to "own" HIV/AIDS because it simply reinforces the stigma already attached to transgenderism, a stigma that their transgenderist political movement is trying to dispel (Bolin, 1994; Feinberg, 1996). Transgender health advocates, including those who represent the most at-risk members of the transgender community, have come forward to claim ownership of HIV risk and prevention in Boston, New York, Philadelphia, and elsewhere. AIDS prevention by transgenders for transgenders is the necessary first step in ownership.

NOTES

1. GISST is housed at Beacon Hill Multicultural Psychological Association in Boston.

2. For example, in his keynote address to the 1997 Second New England Transgender Health Conference, organized by Rebecca Durkee, Leslie Feinberg, a

well-known female-to-male transgender "warrior" and author (1993, 1996), recounted a saga of withheld and inappropriate care that almost cost his life (Gray, 1997, p. A28).

Female-to-male transgenders also face HIV risks. Social stigma and its internalization as low self-esteem contribute to their risks, just as they do to male-to-females' risks. Partly because their hormonal transition is more complete, female-to-male transgenders often pass more easily than their male-to-female sisters (Griggs, 1998, pp. 9, 24). Whereas for male-to-female transgenders hormone replacement therapy does not raise the voice or eliminate the need for electrolysis, for female-to-male transgenders it lowers the voice and encourages facial and body hair growth. American gender ideology may also be a factor in the relative ease of passing, since short men attract less notice than tall women. Greater ease of passing together with the gendered wage gap between males and females in the United States make female-to-male transgenders somewhat less economically vulnerable overall, though individual cases by no means always follow this general rule. A key risk for male-to-female transgenders is participation in prostitution, yet there is no market for female-to-male sex workers. Contributing to female-to-male transgenders' risks, however, is the sexual drive, sometimes both precipitous and strong, brought on by the use of male hormones to effect bodily transition, perhaps accentuated, as Griggs (1998, p. 34) notes, by "cultural reinforcement of masculine [sexual] expression."

3. Many transgenders feel that their contribution to gay liberation is either unacknowledged or insufficiently acknowledged. In 1969, at Stonewall in New York City's Greenwich Village, drag queens and transgenders "fought back against a police bar raid" (Feinberg, 1996, p. 9). Transgenders and drag queens who were thus at the forefront at the Stonewall Rebellion, which is commonly considered the beginning of the gay rights movement, have felt pushed aside, even rejected, by the gay movement in its attempts to gain social and political respectability.

4. For example, the article "Providing Sensitive Health Care to Gay and Lesbian Youth" observes that for those adolescents who do not accept their homosexuality "[i]t is still premature to label during this time of identity development" (Sanford, 1989, p. 35). Another article on the same topic observes that "the 12-year-old boy who has physical and emotional attractions only to other males may question his identity as a male until he feels more secure and healthy about his gay sexual orientation" (Nelson, 1997, p. 106). Interestingly, a sensitive service provider could misconstrue a male-to-female adolescent's female gender self-identity as a lack of self-acceptance of homosexuality.

REFERENCES

ActionAIDS (1994). "Don't Forget HIV/AIDS" (brochure). ActionAIDS: Philadelphia.

Bockting, Walter O., Rosser, B.R. Simon, and Coleman, Eli (1993). *Transgender HIV-AIDS Prevention Program: Manual.* Minneapolis: Program in Human Sexuality, Department of Family Practice and Community Health, Medical School,

University of Minnesota, in collaboration with City of Lakes Crossgender Community, Minnesota Freedom of Gender Expression, Minnesota AIDS Project, and Aliveness Aware.

Bolin, Anne (1988). *In Search of Eve: Transsexual Rites of Passage.* New York: Bergin and Garvey.

Bolin, Anne (1994). "Transcending and Transgendering: Male-to-Female Transsexuals, Dichotomy, and Diversity." In Gilbert Herdt, ed., Third Sex, Third Gender: Beyond Sexual Dimorphism in Culture and History, pp. 447-486. New York: Zone Books.

Durkee, Rebecca Capri (1995). *The Invisible Community—Transgenders and HIV Risks: Training Curriculum.* Boston: Gender Identity Support Services for Transgenders.

Feinberg, Leslie (1993). *Stone Butch Blues.* Ithaca, NY: Firebrand Books.

Feinberg, Leslie (1996). *Transgender Warriors: Making History from Joan of Arc to RuPaul.* Boston: Beacon Press.

Gray, Steven (1997). "Conference Explores Health Care Bias Against Transsexuals." *Boston Globe,* June 4, p. A28.

Green, Jamison, with Brinkin, Larry, and HRC Staff (1994). *Investigation into Discrimination Against Transgendered People.* San Francisco: Human Rights Commission, City and County of San Francisco.

Griggs, Claudine (1998). *S/he: Changing Sex and Changing Clothes.* Oxford: Berg.

Lockett, Gloria (1995). "CAL-PEP: The Struggle to Survive." In Beth E. Schneider and Nancy E. Stoller, eds., *Women Resisting AIDS: Feminist Strategies of Empowerment,* pp. 208-218. Philadelphia: Temple University.

Mason, Theresa Hope, Connors, Margaret M., and Kammerer, Cornelia Ann (1995). *Transgenders and HIV Risks: Needs Assessment.* Boston: Gender Identity Support Services for Transgenders, prepared for the Massachusetts Department of Public Health HIV/AIDS Bureau.

Nelson, John A. (1997). "Gay, Lesbian, and Bisexual Adolescents: Providing Esteem-Enhancing Care to a Battered Population." *The Nurse Practitioner* 22(2), pp. 94-109.

Newton, Esther (1972). *Mother Camp: Female Impersonation in America.* Englewood Cliffs, NJ: Prentice-Hall.

PWAC of New York (1996). "AIDS in the Transgender Community," *Newsline,* April, pp. 6-38.

Raymond, Janice G. (1994 [1979]). *The Transsexual Empire: The Making of the She-Male.* New York: Teachers College Press.

Rothblatt, Martine (1995). *The Apartheid of Sex: A Manifesto on the Freedom of Gender.* New York: Crown Publishers.

Sanford, Nancy D. (1989). "Providing Sensitive Health Care to Gay and Lesbian Youth." *The Nurse Practitioner* 14(5), pp. 30-47.

Stuart, Kim Elizabeth (1991). *The Uninvited Dilemma: A Question of Gender.* Portland, OR: Metamorphous Press.

Valentine, David (forthcoming). " 'We're Not About Gender': How an Emerging Transgender Movement Challenges Gay and Lesbian Theory to Put the 'Gender'

Back into 'Sexuality.'" In Bill Leap and Ellen Lewin, eds. *Anthropology Comes Out: Lesbians, Gays, Cultures.* Urbana, IL: University of Illinois Press.

Withers, Kristine (1995). "Notes from a Survivor," *LAP Notes* 3, p. 12. New York: Lesbian AIDS Project of the Gay Men's Health Crisis.

Woodhouse, Annie (1989). *Fantastic Women: Sex, Gender, and Transvestism.* New Brunswick, NJ: Rutgers University Press.

Chapter 4

HIV Risk Behaviors of Male-to-Female Transgenders in a Community-Based Harm Reduction Program

Cathy J. Reback
Emilia L. Lombardi

OVERVIEW OF THE COMMUNITY-BASED PROGRAM

The Van Ness Recovery House and Van Ness Prevention Division

The Van Ness Recovery House is a nonprofit corporation dedicated to serving the needs of gay, lesbian, bisexual, and transgender/transsexual substance users. The recovery house, which was founded in 1973, is a ninety-day, twenty-bed residential drug and alcohol treatment facility. The Van Ness Recovery House served its first transgendered resident in 1984. Between 1984 and 1988, the Van Ness Recovery House served one to two transgendered residents per year.

This research was funded by Contract No. H208837-2 from the U.S. Centers for Disease Control and Prevention and the County of Los Angeles Department of Health Services' Office of AIDS Programs and Policy. Dr. Reback would like to thank the field staff of the Van Ness Recovery House Prevention Division for their ongoing commitment and hard work and Kathleen Watt for her support of this program. Dr. Lombardi would like to thank Talia Bettcher, Shirley Bushnell, and Jacob Hale.

Correspondence and requests for materials can be sent to Cathy J. Reback, PhD, 1136 N. La Brea Avenue, West Hollywood, California 90038, <Rebackcj@aol.com>.

Since 1988 to present, the Van Ness Recovery House has consistently served from ten to twenty transgendered residents per year. Additionally, since 1988, we have had a minimum of one transgendered person on staff.

In December 1994, the Van Ness Recovery House began its Prevention Division, which offers HIV and substance abuse prevention interventions to gay, lesbian, bisexual, and transgender/transsexual drug users in the Hollywood and West Hollywood areas of California. The Van Ness Prevention Division (VNPD) is based on the philosophy of harm reduction. The overall objective of the prevention programs is to reduce the harm that can result from drug use by preventing HIV infection and managing the physical, psychological, and psychosocial manifestations of drug use without the requirement of abstinence or recovery. Success is evaluated by any change in behavior that reduces physical, psychological, or psychosocial harm to our participants, their loved ones, and/or their communities.

VNPD staff conduct face-to-face street outreach, counseling interventions, immediate linkage to services, pre-and posttest counseling, education/prevention groups, community workshops, art exploration groups, and support groups. These services are provided on the streets in identified high-risk areas of Hollywood, in natural settings where participants congregate (including street corners, bars, fast-food stands, parks, bathhouses, and sex clubs) and at the Prevention Division site located at the intersection of the Hollywood and West Hollywood stroll districts.

The Transgender Harm Reduction Program

The VNPD Transgender Harm Reduction Program was initiated in October 1996 and is designed to reach a variety of male-to-female (MTF) transgendered individuals, including persons living on the streets or in low-rent hotels, sex workers, bar queens, as well as those integrated and living in the suburbs. The program defines an MTF transgender as an individual who was born male but identifies as a woman. These transgendered women may be at different stages in their social role transition from man to woman.

The specific prevention interventions offered are based on a needs assessment done prior to program implementation that included in-depth interviews and a focus group with members of the target population. Efforts are made to have repeated contacts with clients to enhance trust and encourage participation in the community workshops and mentoring support group.

The workshop topics include grooming and hygiene, legalization and documentation, health care, and hormone therapy. These areas were chosen based on the results of the needs assessment. The program consists of an outreach component and a series of four community workshops designed to promote skills building and behavior change to reduce HIV risk, a weekly mentoring support group, and job training. Implicit in each workshop topic is the importance of increasing self-esteem as an important precursor for adopting safer behavior. Each workshop also includes an explicit HIV/AIDS risk reduction component. Concurrent with the community workshops is the weekly mentoring support group. The format of the support group is open, thereby providing an opportunity for participants to choose the topic for discussion. The program participants who complete the four community workshops and maintain ongoing participation in the support group are encouraged to serve as mentors to the newer participants. Job training is available to each participant after completing the four community workshops. Participants are also referred for HIV counseling and testing and other services as needed.

METHOD

During the first eighteen months of the program, January 1996 through June 1997, 861 MTF transgender/transsexual persons were contacted through street outreach. Of those, 209 participated in the Transgender Harm Reduction Program. Demographic data were collected during the first outreach contact, and a more in-depth HIV risk assessment, including drug and sex behaviors, was conducted at a baseline intervention session. Follow-up risk assessments were conducted at each subsequent intervention session.

Analysis

Data from the 209 intervention participants were analyzed by comparing individuals who reported exchanging sex for money and/or drugs sometime in the previous thirty days with those who did not. Analysis of variance was conducted upon demographic factors such as age, ethnicity, marginal living situation (living in a low-rent hotel, rooming house, or shelter, or on the streets), and whether they were monolingual

Spanish speakers. The difference in substance use was assessed by identifying which substances were used by the intervention participants. Finally, differences in sexual activity were analyzed by identifying the number of exchange and nonexchange male sexual partners the participants reported within the previous thirty days and the percentage of reported condom use during these sexual encounters.

Demographics

Of the 209 participants in the Transgender Harm Reduction Program, 40 percent were Latin/Hispanic, 28 percent Caucasian, 22 percent African American, 6 percent Asian/Pacific Islander, 3 percent Native American, and 1 percent multiracial or other. Their ages ranged from sixteen to fifty-five years, and the mean age was thirty-one years. Of the participants, 26 percent reported a marginal or transitional living situation at the baseline intervention, such as a low-rent hotel (13 percent); on the streets (5 percent), for example, "squatting" in an abandoned building, finding shelter in a vacant lot or abandoned car, or sleeping in a park; or living in a shelter or other service facility (2 percent). Of the participants, 79 percent identified as heterosexual, 10 percent as bisexual, 8 percent as gay, and 2 percent as lesbian (see Table 4.1). Sexual identity takes on varied meanings within transgender communities and must be considered when creating transgender-specific programs. For example, an HIV intervention participant could be an MTF transgender who identifies as lesbian and has a penis.

Alcohol and Drug Use

Table 4.2 summarizes the extent of drug and alcohol use by participants in the previous thirty days. At the baseline intervention, almost half (45 percent) of the participants reported some alcohol and/or drug use in the previous thirty days. Alcohol was the most frequently used substance by the program participants, with 37 percent reporting use, and 13 percent reported using marijuana at least once in the previous thirty days. The third most frequently used drugs were crack and crystal methamphetamine, with 11 percent of the participants using each in the previous thirty days. Of the participants, 7 percent reported cocaine use and 2 percent reported heroin use within the time period measured (see Table 4.2).

TABLE 4.1. Demographic Characteristics of Program Participants (N = 209)

Variable	Percentage
Age:	
<20	7.2
21-29	45.9
30-39	28.2
>39	18.7
Mean age = 30.7	
Race/ethnicity:	
Latin/Hispanic	40.2
Caucasian	28.2
African American	21.5
Asian/Pacific Islander	6.2
Native American	2.9
Multiracial or other	1.0
Monolingual Spanish speakers	10.8
Homeless or marginal living situation	25.5
Sexual identity:	
Heterosexual	79.0
Bisexual	10.2
Gay	8.3
Lesbian	2.4

TABLE 4.2. Drug Use of Program Participants (N = 209)

Drug Use in Previous Thirty Days	Percentage
Alcohol	37.0
Marijuana	12.5
Crack	11.1
Crystal	11.1
Cocaine	7.2
Heroin	1.9

Approximately 5 percent of the participants reported injection drug use in the previous thirty days, as seen in Table 4.3. The most frequently injected drug was crystal methamphetamine (4 percent), and only a few individuals reported injecting either cocaine or heroin. Only a small proportion of those within the intervention were at risk of HIV infection due to injection drug use. Of those reporting any in-

TABLE 4.3. Injection Drug Use and Risks (N = 209)*

Injection Drug Use	Percentage
Any injection drug use	4.5
Crystal	4.0
Heroin	2.0
Cocaine	1.0

*Multiple responses were possible

jection use in the previous thirty days, only one-third reported using a needle exchange program or bleach to clean their needles, and twenty percent reported never sharing needles.

Sex Work

Baseline data from the 209 program participants were analyzed by comparing those who reported sex work (n = 76) with those who did not (n = 133). Although 44 percent identified as sex workers at outreach contact, at the baseline intervention session only 36 percent reported exchanging sex for money and/or drugs in the previous thirty days.

The differences between sex workers and non-sex workers are summarized in Table 4.4. The mean age of sex workers was younger than for non-sex workers (26.9 versus 32.9). Sex workers were more likely than non-sex workers to be Latin/Hispanic (60.5 versus 28.6 percent), were significantly less likely to be Caucasian (10.5 versus 38.4 percent), and equally likely to be African American (21.8 versus 21.1 percent). Among the Latin/Hispanic transgenders in the program, those who engaged in sex work were more likely to be monolingual Spanish speakers (18.4 versus 7.5 percent). Additionally, sex workers were significantly more likely to be homeless or to live marginally than non-sex workers (42.1 versus 14.6 percent).

Sex work was also associated with greater substance use. Those who engaged in sex work were significantly more likely to report alcohol use in the previous thirty days (51 versus 29 percent), marijuana use (20 versus 8 percent), crack use (25 versus 3 percent), crystal use (21 versus 5 percent), and cocaine use (12 versus 5 percent). Additionally, sex workers were significantly more likely to be injectors than

TABLE 4.4. Comparison Between Sex Workers and Non-Sex Workers (Percent) (N = 209)

	Sex Workers (N = 76)	Non-Sex Workers (N = 133)
Mean age	26.9	32.9
Homeless or marginal living situation	42.1%	14.6%**
Race/ethnicity		
African-American	21.1%	21.8%
Caucasian	10.5%	38.3%**
Latin/Hispanic	60.6%	28.6%**
Asian	3.9%	7.5%
Native American	3.9%	2.3%
Multiracial or other	0	1.5%
Alcohol use	51.3%	28.8%**
Crack use	25.0%	3.0%**
Crystal use	21.1%	5.3%**
Marijuana use	19.7%	8.3%*
Cocaine use	11.8%	4.5%*
Injection drug use	9.2%	2.3%*
Injected crystal	7.9%	1.5%*
Injected heroin	3.9%	0.7%
Number of times with male sex partner	20.9	2.6**
Condom use during sex with male partner	94.3%	55.6%**
Number of times performed sex work	28.5	0
Condom use during sex work	95.3%	0

*p = .05
**p = .001

non-sex workers (9 versus 2 percent); this also included injecting crystal (8 versus 2 percent). In a recent study of methamphetamine use, the transgender respondents reported using the drug to enhance sexual encounters during sex work (Reback, 1997).

There are also differences between sex workers and non-sex workers in their sexual activity with nonexchange male partners. Those engaged in sex work reported having a greater number of nonexchange male sexual partners (21 versus 3) in the previous thirty days. However, the sex workers demonstrated greater understanding of HIV transmission risks as well as a greater personal perception of risk, as is evidenced in their reported condom use. Sex workers reported a high use of condoms with their exchange partners (95 percent) and were more likely to use condoms with their nonexchange male sex partners than non-sex workers (94 versus 56 percent). Consequently, among this sample, although sex workers reported significantly more male partners, their HIV risk through sexual behavior may be lower than for non-sex workers as a result of their higher use of condoms.

CONCLUSION AND DISCUSSION

Little is known about the HIV risks of MTF transgendered persons, although past studies have found a high HIV seroprevalence rate among MTF transgendered women (Simon, Reback, and Bemis, in press; Sykes, 1999; Pang, Pugh, and Catalan, 1994; Rekart, Manzon, and Tucker, 1993; Modan et al., 1992; Alan, Guinan, and McCallum, 1989). One of the primary reasons given for their high rate of HIV infection has been the high prevalence of sex work among the individuals within their samples (Simon, Reback, and Bemis, n.d.). We also found a similar pattern within these data. Those who exchanged sex were found to use more drugs and alcohol, including more injection drug use, than those not engaged in sex work. In addition to their exchange sex partners, the sex workers reported a greater number of nonexchange male sex partners. However, the sex workers reported greater condom use than non-sex workers.

Past studies on transgender HIV risk factors have focused primarily on individual risk factors and have not dealt with the social context that could influence one's individual risk factors. It is possible that the marginalization of these individuals creates a social context that places them at risk of HIV infection. For example, Sanjay (1996) concludes that much of the HIV risk experienced by transsexuals in India was due to their illegal status and, consequently, their limited access to legal and social resources. A similar situation exists in the United States. For MTF transgenders, a legal identity that is inconsistent with one's presenting gender may lead to employment discrimination, which serves to drive many into illegal forms of employment. Boles and Elifson (1994) also note a relationship between transgender discrimination and sex work.

For transgendered persons, it is often difficult and costly to establish a legal identity in one's chosen gender. The inconsistency between one's legal gender identity and gender presentation may force many transgendered persons into the margins of society. For many, this marginalization forces them into work that does not require legal documentation. Of the participants in the Transgender Harm Reduction Program, 55 percent of those who were Latin/Hispanic and 58 percent of those who were monolingual Spanish speakers engaged in sex work. Furthermore, the current political climate for all undocumented immigrants in California creates difficulty in gaining legal documentation.

Transgendered persons currently have little protection from discrimination in the workplace. A previous study found 37 percent of the sample reported some type of employment or economic discrimination, such as not being hired or losing one's job due to one's presenting gender (GenderPAC, 1997). Employment discrimination may force people into sex work due to the limited choices given to transgendered persons.

Another employment consideration is job accessibility. For many undocumented women, access to domestic jobs such as child care and other housework services is usually obtained through family support networks, and many transgendered women are estranged from their families. The lack of access to jobs could serve to pressure transgendered women into sex work.

The data from this study came from a community-based HIV harm reduction program. Given that only a limited amount of data can be collected prior to an intervention session, both the contact and intervention forms must be brief. Therefore, information was collected on participants' current drug use and sexual behaviors. Further studies are needed to examine the legal, social, and economic situations of transgendered persons.

REFERENCES

Alan, D.L., J. Guinan, and L. McCallum (1989). "HIV Seroprevalence and Its Implications for a Transsexual Population." *V International Conference on AIDS*, 5:748.

Boles, J. and K.W. Elifson (1994). "The Social Organization of Transvestite Prostitution and AIDS." *Social Science and Medicine* 39(1):85-93.

GenderPAC (1997). *First National Survey of Transgender Violence*. New York: GenderPAC.

Modan, B., Goldschmidt, R., Rubinstein, E. Vonsover, A., Zinn, M., Golan, R., Chetrit, A., Gottlieb-Stematzkyk, T. (1992). "Prevalence of HIV Antibodies in Transsexual and Female Prostitutes." *American Journal of Public Health*, 82(4):590-592.

Pang, H., K. Pugh, and J. Catalan (1994). "Gender Identity Disorder and HIV Disease." *International Journal of STD and AIDS,* 5(2):130-132.

Reback, C.J. (1997). *The Social Construction of a Gay Drug: Methamphetamine Use Among Gay and Bisexual Males in Los Angeles.* (Report for the City of Los Angeles, AIDS Coordinator). Los Angeles: Author.

Rekart, M.L., L.M. Manzon, and P. Tucker (1993). "Transsexuals and AIDS." *IX International Conference on AIDS,* 9:734.

Sanjay, G. (1996). "HIV/AIDS Intervention Among Transsexuals in Bangalore, Medico-Legal Impediments for Effective Intervention." *XI International Conference on AIDS,* 11:52.

Simon, P., C.J. Reback, and C. Bemis (n.d.). HIV Risk Profile of an Urban Transgender Population. Unpublished manuscript.

Simon, P., C.J. Reback, and C. Bemis (in press). "HIV Prevalence and Incidence Among Male-to-Female Transgenders Receiving HIV Prevention Services in Los Angeles County." *AIDS.*

Sykes, D.L. (1999). "Transgendered People: An 'Invisible' Population." *California HIV/AIDS Update,* 12(1):80-85.

Chapter 5

HIV Prevention
and Health Service Needs
of the Transgender Community
in San Francisco

Kristen Clements-Nolle
Willy Wilkinson
Kerrily Kitano
Rani Marx

BACKGROUND

Previous research suggests that transgendered persons in the United States are at high risk for acquiring HIV. A small study of transgendered sex workers in Atlanta found that 68 percent were seropositive for HIV,

The authors would like to acknowledge the work of the Transgender Advisory Committee members (Connie Amarthitada, Neil Broome, Tamara Ching, Russell Hilkene, Jade Kwan, Yosenio Lewis, Margaret Morvay, Major, Gina Tucker, Adela Vasquez, and Kiki Whitlock), the Department of Public Health AIDS Office staff (Celinda Cantu, Gene Copello, Veronica Davila, Brian Dobrow, Delia Garcia, Keiko Kim, Michael Pendo, Tracey Packer, and Billy Pick), and our focus group transcriber (Marilyn McDonald).

A special thanks to the agencies and their clients who made this project possible: Asian AIDS Project (now known as the Asian and Pacific Islander Wellness Center), Brothers Network (now known as New Village), the Center for Special Problems, the Center for Southeast Asian Refugee Resettlement (now known as Southeast Asian Community Center), Proyecto ContraSIDA Por Vida, San Francisco County Jail (San Bruno), Tenderloin AIDS Resource Center, and the Tom Waddell Clinic.

Correspondence and requests for materials should be sent to Kristen Clements-Nolle, MPH, San Francisco Department of Public Health, AIDS Office, 25 Van Ness Avenue, Suite #500, San Francisco, California, 94102; Tel: (415)554-9496; e-mail-<kristen-clements@dph.sf.ca.us>.

69

81 percent had seromarkers for syphilis, and 80 percent had seromarkers for hepatitis B.[1] The prevalence of HIV infection in this population was much higher than for nontransgendered sex workers in the same neighborhoods.[2] A study with a more representative sample of the transgender community found that 15 percent of transgendered individuals seeking hormone therapy at a San Francisco public health clinic were infected with HIV.[3] Qualitative studies conducted in Minneapolis, Boston, Los Angeles, and San Francisco provide further evidence that many transgendered persons engage in behaviors that may put them at risk for HIV, such as injection drug use and commercial sex work.[4-8] These qualitative studies also identify psychosocial factors, such as low socioeconomic status, social isolation, and low self-esteem, that are probably associated with risk-taking behaviors.

Although important studies, a number of limitations characterize this prior research. To date, all studies have focused almost exclusively on male-to-female (MTF) populations, despite anecdotal evidence that suggests many female-to-male (FTM) transgendered individuals are also at risk for HIV infection (from injecting hormones and having unprotected anal sex with gay men). In addition, past studies have sampled a very small number of individuals (often fewer than twenty), limiting the analysis and generalizability of findings.

We conducted eleven focus groups with a large (N = 100) and diverse population of MTF and FTM transgendered persons in San Francisco to assess their HIV risk and access to HIV prevention and health services. We found high rates of HIV risk behaviors such as unprotected sex, commercial sex work, and injection drug use. Participants cited low self-esteem, substance abuse, and economic necessity as common barriers to adopting and maintaining safer behaviors. Participants also stated that competing priorities, fear of discrimination, and the insensitivity of service providers were the primary factors that keep them, and other transgendered people they know, from accessing HIV prevention and health services. Participants' recommendations for improving services include hiring transgendered persons to develop and implement programs and training existing providers in transgender sensitivity and standards of care.

METHODS

Sampling

From June 24 to August 8, 1996, ten focus groups were conducted at agencies with existing services for the transgender population and one group was held in a San Francisco county jail. Of the eleven groups, one was African American, one, Latina bilingual, one, Latina monolingual, two, primarily Asian and Pacific Islander, and one, FTM. The remaining groups were composed of both MTF and FTM participants of various racial/ethnic identities. Subjects were recruited primarily by HIV prevention agency staff who had extensive experience working with the transgender community in San Francisco. Many subjects had accessed the participating agency's services previously or had some contact with the agency staff.

Procedures

Each group was facilitated by a trained Department of Public Health (DPH) staff person and a member of the transgender community. The facilitators all followed a standardized outline and set of questions. Participants were asked to respond as a group to questions that addressed access to and use of HIV prevention and health services in San Francisco (see Table 5.1). Each participant was given a list of specific prevention interventions and health care services available in San Francisco to ensure that everyone understood service terminology. Although participants were not directly asked about HIV risk behaviors, discussion of sex work, drug use, and unprotected sex was frequent in each of the focus group sessions. Participants were assured complete anonymity and were told that disclosure of HIV status was voluntary. However, it is clear from self-disclosure that individuals living with HIV were represented in most of the focus groups.

TABLE 5.1. Focus Group Questions

- What types of HIV prevention activities have you (or your clients) participated in?
- What did you like and/or dislike about these prevention activities or services?
- If you could design your own HIV prevention program, what would you do to keep the transgendered people you know from getting infected with HIV?
- What types of health services have you or anyone you know used?
- What has been your experience (or others' experiences) with these services?
- What would you suggest doing to improve health services for people in your community who are infected with HIV?
- What do you think we could do to reach transgendered persons who are not currently coming to agencies and clinics for prevention activities or health services?

After the focus groups were completed, participants were given a twenty-dollar stipend and asked to complete a short, anonymous questionnaire that assessed their demographics. All focus groups were professionally taped by a transcriber who took notes during the discussion and numbered the responses of different individuals. The monolingual Spanish group was transcribed by a Spanish-speaking transcriber and translated by a Spanish-speaking DPH staff person.

Coding and Analysis

The focus group transcripts were read and coded separately by two researchers trained in qualitative analysis. Participants' comments were coded into twenty-eight categories that naturally emerged from the data in the following areas: (1) HIV risk behaviors, (2) factors associated with HIV risk behaviors, (3) HIV prevention interventions, and (4) HIV/AIDS-related services. Comments were transcribed verbatim and assigned to the appropriate category; they were cross-referenced if they addressed more than one category. Within categories, only comments from unduplicated individuals were enumerated. For example, if one participant made several comments about a particular issue or category, those comments were counted collectively as one. Participant comments (unduplicated) that indicated agreement with a previous comment were counted in the same category as the original participant comment. The topic areas and quotes highlighted in this manuscript are those with the highest number of unduplicated comments.

Comments about HIV prevention activities and HIV/AIDS-related services were counted if they indicated *unmet* need (i.e., need for improved services or needing but not getting a service). Though many comments described participants' use and awareness of prevention interventions and HIV/AIDS-related services, we did not include them in this analysis.

RESULTS

Sociodemographics

One hundred individuals participated in the eleven focus groups. Almost two-thirds of the sample were nonwhite, 29 percent of the sample were born in countries outside the United States, and 28 percent reported that they usually speak a language other than English (see Table 5.2). Participants ranged in age from eighteen to sixty-six years; the average age was thirty-five. Most of the sample was male-to-female (82 percent) and self-identified as either straight or bisexual/pansexual.

TABLE 5.2. Demographic Characteristics of 100 Transgendered Focus Group Participants

Characteristic	Percentage (N = 100)
Age Range 18-66 years **Mean Range** 34.7 years	
Race/Ethnicity	
White	37
Latino/Hispanic	24
African American	16
Asian or Pacific Islander*	11
Mixed race/multiethnic	9
Native American	3
Nativity/Country of Origin	
American born	70
Foreign born	29
Missing	1
Gender Identification	
Transgender (MTF)	65
Female (born male)	12
Transsexual (MTF)	5
Transgender (FTM)	7
Male (born female)	3
Intersexed	2
Other	4
Missing	2
Sexual Orientation	
Straight/heterosexual	38
Bisexual/pansexual	22
Gay/homosexual	19
Other	12
Lesbian	5
Missing	4

*Asian and Pacific Islander category included. Chinese, Filipino, Hawaiian, Laotian, and Vietnamese.

HIV Risk Behaviors

Sex Work

Although no focus group questions specifically addressed sex work, this issue was discussed at length in all of the focus groups except the FTM group. Many focus group participants had engaged in sex work at some point in their lives and discussed sex work as a pervasive issue in their communities. Participants named economic necessity as the main reason for personal and community involvement in sex work. It was commonly stated that sex work, or "survival sex," was the only option for many transgendered people because of the severe job, housing, and education discrimination that they face. Participants also observed a strong association between drug use (particularly methamphetamine use) and sex work. Some participants said they use drugs to "deal with" sex work, and others stated that they engage in sex work to support their drug addiction.

> The whole scenario of prostitution in our TG community is . . . I wish we could be treated like anybody else and have the same job opportunities as anybody else . . . and I wouldn't have to go stand on the damn street. I'm a very intelligent person.

> I'm on SSI, and I make almost $800 a month. I have a college education. I've owned nightclubs, restaurants. I've been an actor. I've been a professional all my life. But my choices now are to be on SSI disability and prostitute. I guess some girls can find jobs, but there's a lot of prejudice out there.

> I know I have a little bit of money saved up. But that's gonna run out sooner or later, so I have to go back to my original support. And so I'm really taking a chance by doing that. Which I know is wrong, but I'm not gonna starve either.

> Most of the time it comes down to a couple of things. Number one, it's economics. People are on drugs, and that's the only way they can make money to get drugs. Number two, there's a fatalism aspect.

Participants frequently described a cyclic pattern of engaging in sex work, being incarcerated, and returning to sex work upon release due to lack of employment opportunities. Many individuals who were currently in jail or had recently been incarcerated stated that they were HIV positive and desperately wanted to obtain job training and education to get out of sex work. However, the barriers to getting such training were so great that they did not feel they would ever break out of the pattern of prostitution and incarceration.

> I cannot go to school because I'm HIV positive, and I'm going to end up being a prostitute again, get arrested, lose my apartment. If I sell my body or use drugs, I don't have my self-esteem . . this whole circle.

> All the girls that I know about, when they have HIV, they have nothin' goin' for themselves whatsoever. When they get out of jail, only thing they have to do is resort back to prostitution and come back in here again! When you have HIV, and you did nothin' for your entire life but prostitution, what is there else to do?

> I was tested in court, and I came out positive. The judge told me that I would either stop prostituting or would have to serve the time in prison. But they don't have anything to help. They should have some kind of group or program that could point out my alternatives.

Another rationale given by participants for pervasive prostitution in the transgender community was validation of one's gender identity, though this was less frequently mentioned than economic necessity. For many MTF participants, being paid to have sex as a female (usually by heterosexually identified clients) reinforced their gender identity and boosted their self-esteem.

> There's something about the glamour of being on the stroll. It's fast, easy money. Shake your tits, shake your tush, and have some guy slip you twenty, fifty, a hundred dollars. It builds up your self-esteem!

> Oh, somebody's paying them, so they must look real, that validates their femininity.

There are a lot of TGs that have jobs, making twenty, thirty, forty thousand dollars, but they still go to the [bar] and prostitute, because it builds their self-esteem.

Unprotected Sex

In all of the focus groups, participants spoke about their own unsafe sexual behavior and unsafe sex that occurs within their communities. Both MTF and FTM participants stated that low self-esteem was the main reason for sexual risk taking. Many participants mentioned that passing, or being accepted sexually as male or female, often contributes to self-esteem and willingness to engage in unprotected sex and other high-risk behaviors. Participants also explained that society's view of the transgender community takes an enormous toll on their self-esteem and can contribute to self-destructive behavior.

> When you have a low self-esteem and this fine guy comes up to you and it's like, "I want to have sex with you," and he's so fine, and you're like, "If I want to use a condom, he's not gonna want to do it!"

> I went out with a guy who I knew was HIV positive, and I had unsafe sex with him because he showed attraction for me. There's a part of me that's self-destructive. I mean, you know, we don't really seem to matter! I mean, we put all this work into looking like women. We do all this stuff . . . and it still isn't good enough.

> I've been in risky sexual situations just for the attention actually, or just for the acceptance as being male.

> For those of us who aren't prostitutes, if we get recognition by a man as being a woman, sometimes you just grab onto that, and maybe ordinarily you would be cautious. In a case like that, you just let it all out, 'cause someone's accepting you as female.

FTM participants felt that engaging in unprotected sex was a part of exploring one's new gender identity. Many participants acknowledged a disassociation between their gender identity and their physical bodies. This disassociation and denial about engaging in certain types of sexual behaviors (i.e., an FTM who denies he has vaginal sex) are barriers to engaging in protected sex. Many FTM participants also felt that testosterone use increased their sex drive and the sexual risks they were willing to take. Several FTMs also said they started to have sexual relations with men, rather than women, after they started hormone therapy.

> I've visited some of the glory hole areas of the city. I have felt like it's a place I can go and experience sex with other men, where I don't have to worry about . . . are they gonna read me as female?

> For gay FTMs, we might be willing to do something with some- one that's less than safe because it's like, "Oh my God, an op- portunity to have this gay experience." I feel that.

> My sex drive is totally different now (with testosterone use). It puts me in more of a head space where I'm more likely to do riskier activities than I would've done before.

> There's less of a connection between our identities and our physical bodies. We behave in ways sexually and take risks that maybe you wouldn't think would fit our identity.

MTF participants who engaged in sex work typically stated that they were more likely to use condoms with "johns" than with their husbands, boyfriends, and nonpaying sex partners. However, many stated that they have unprotected sex with clients if they are paid more to do so. Some also stated that if they insisted on condom use, they could be physically abused by their clients.

> This city is so full of ignorance along these issues that a lot of girls . . . feel like there's nothin' else they can do. They can't even do the community college when it's free because of the stigma, so they wind up doing sex work. And they're out there, and, yes, they want to use condoms, but goddammit, if they've gotta make rent . . . if they've gotta keep somebody who expects something happy . . . if they want to eat, if they want their drugs . . .

> I'm asymptomatic . . . but it's hard when dates think I look cute, and that I don't look like I've got AIDS, and they don't want to use a condom, and if it's a three hundred-dollar date, I'm like, "Screw it" and then I have unprotected sex with them anyways.

Remember, you are hungry, you haven't had anything for a couple of days, and this jerk comes up and says, "I have twenty dollars, and I don't want to use a condom." What are you gonna do? You're gonna take his twenty dollars, and you're gonna deal with this freak. Sometimes they put you in a situation that you say, "I have to do this because this freak might come back and really attack me."

Alcohol and Drug Use

Although no specific questions about substance use were asked, discussion of frequent injection and noninjection drug use in the transgender community did take place. Several individuals believed they became infected with HIV from sharing syringes. Participants thought that the prevalence of drug use in their respective communities was a result of lack of education and job opportunities, low self-esteem, and limited social support. As stated previously, participants believed that drug addiction and prostitution often coincide and are mutually reinforcing.

I'm shooting up on heroin. I'm shooting up on speed. I been using one needle for almost a week, and they say that's how I got HIV.

A lot of the transsexuals I know who are prostitutes are having unprotected sex and they're also shooting up . . . and sharing needles.

A lot of FTMs in the community are struggling with drug and alcohol issues, and there is no inpatient or really adequate outpatient treatment to meet the needs of FTMs.

It's about the self-esteem issue. You feel like, at times, that you're doomed to live your life all by yourself, and that plays into HIV status, 'cause you figure, "What the fuck? I might as well go ahead and go out and have a good time, and die from it. I might as well get loaded. What does it matter?"

I have a girlfriend . . . at one time she was the most beautifulest [sic] woman in the world. Now she's livin' in a hotel and smokin' crack! And that's the only thing she talks about! "Please give me hit!" It's because she has no support.

HIV Prevention and Health Service Barriers

Competing Priorities

HIV was not a primary concern for many participants. Participants generally agreed that securing employment, housing, and substance abuse/mental health treatment were more pressing issues for many transgendered people, and that such issues had to be addressed before HIV prevention and/or treatment would be effective. Participants underscored the need for transgender-specific job training, job placement, housing placement, and substance abuse/mental health programs, including transgender sensitivity training for landlords, employers, and service providers.

> Not looking at these other issues like employment that are not related directly to AIDS prevention is an unwise thing to do. I think these things are all very interrelated and interdependent. And they have to be addressed.

> If you get the people off the drugs and the alcohol . . . you're gonna cut down on both the STDs and AIDS. And I'll tell you right now that there is not a truly transgender-friendly recovery program in this city.

> If it's anything that pushes me . . . into tough, bad things, like drugs or coming up close with AIDS, it's the unemployment thing.

> There are a lot of girls that are sex workers because they have no choice. It's pure survival. And we're in desperate need of training and education, to upgrade our skills, and then find employers who will employ us. And in terms of long-term prevention, if you cut down the number of sex workers, you're gonna cut down AIDS, so I see job training as vital.

> Housing and employment are the biggest issues for our community. There's major discrimination through building owners. It took me four months to find an apartment that would accept me, besides roach coaches.

Sensitivity of Providers

Participants in all of the focus groups highlighted the insensitivity of service providers as a major barrier to receiving HIV prevention and health services. Participants stated that they often experienced discrimination when they tried to obtain services, particularly from "gay and lesbian" agencies. There was also frequent discussion about providers who make assumptions about gender identity and do not differentiate MTF clients from gay men, or FTM clients from butch lesbians. The FTM participants expressed a great deal of concern that service providers have little knowledge about the FTM population and do not understand their specific needs. Participants generally believed that a transgendered person who has a negative experience when trying to receive services is unlikely to return to the agency or seek other services in the future.

> A lot of the service organizations exclude us. They focus mainly on the lesbian and gay community. I was at an agency, and these gay boys were just coming and going. I waited two hours, and they just forgot about me! I would rather go to a heterosexual organization and get help from them than go to a lesbian and gay organization because, a lot of times, the lesbian and gay community does leave us out.

> Every time I've gotten tested, I've run across people looking at me, deciding that I'm female, or deciding whatever, and then determining what my actions are, without asking me. Don't assume what my activities are based on how you perceive me.

> They [the clinic staff] are up on all of the HIV stuff, but they don't want to see us transgenders there.

> I went to [the clinic] and they refused to treat me as . . . a person, pretty much. I stated that I was transgender, and they still called me by my boy's name, just because it's on the record. And that really causes . . . well, I feel embarrassed. And that makes me reluctant to go back to these services, because of past experience.

> The girls don't feel comfortable going to a male-oriented clinic. I'm not a gay man. I just can't click with that. I'm a transsexual.

I'm a woman. I'm not a man. I may have been born male, but I'm not a man.

They [health care providers] know about MTF issues but not FTM at all.

Unmet Need: HIV Prevention Interventions

Street Outreach

Participants emphasized the value of street-based outreach and education but stated that more outreach activities had to be conducted by outreach workers who are members of the transgender community. Participants suggested that outreach activities need to be expanded in an effort to reach hidden populations such as FTMs and MTF sex workers who advertise their services in papers and do not hang out in the usual bar and street settings. Many of the groups also introduced the idea of tailoring outreach efforts to the male clientele of MTF sex workers, rather than always targeting the sex workers. Overall, there was agreement that outreach workers need to offer all forms of safer-sex information and materials so that assumptions are not made about the sexual behaviors of different transgendered individuals.

We need to create an outreach program and have more of the transgender community trained around issues of HIV and AIDS, where there are stipends, and have the transgenders go out into the community and do the street outreach.

Ways of reaching out to different parts of the community are gonna have to be adaptable to that community. With the FTM community, you're probably gonna have to go where they're at, or it's gonna be like trying to find a needle in a haystack.

Thanks to all these sex ads and newspapers, you know, a lot of the working girls in the community do not go out to bars anymore, so it makes the outreach harder. Because those girls want to stay invisible. The girls that are working out of [newspapers], they don't want to go in for services.

We need to reach and educate the men, the heterosexual-identified male clientele.

Individual Risk Reduction and Education

Participants felt that HIV prevention education for individuals and their partners is very important, but most believed such interventions are not effective because they are not transgender specific. Many participants expressed concern that their gender identification is not addressed in HIV risk reduction education and counseling sessions. MTF individuals discussed the need for counseling and education that builds their self-esteem; FTMs emphasized the need for counseling that directly addresses their new gender and sexual identities.

> Counseling needs to address self-esteem. And there's a lot of girls, and a lot of guys, in the community, that are very low self-esteem . . . because of mainly what has happened to them in the past. And they will latch onto almost anybody that will pay attention to them, especially when they want to be recognized as male or female.

> I would like to see more counseling that addresses gay FTMs in a more direct way.

> There needs to be a sufficient level of safety to talk about things like getting penetrated in your vagina. I'm telling you, we [FTMs] are doing everything with everybody out there—in every possible combination you can imagine. It's important that those identities and those sexual experiences be validated.

HIV Prevention Support Groups

Participants expressed a need for a space where they could talk with their peers about the complex issues and problems that they face. Frequent suggestions for improving support groups included (1) educating individuals about condom use and safe hormone/drug injection, (2) improving self-esteem, (3) developing safer-sex negotiation skills, and (4) helping clients build job skills to facilitate a transition out of commercial sex work. Participants also called for specific groups for FTMs, youth, and those who speak languages other than English.

> The more we talk about this, the more I really am feeling that some kind of support group-type environment would be really

useful for us, to have a space where we can talk about the really specific things that are different from straight genetic men and gay genetic men, the real specific issues around increasing sex drive, and trying to re-create an identity for ourselves as sexual men.

We need more support. I've been attending this support group and it's really good. I'm at risk, you know. I'm badly on drugs, and really didn't care about anybody or myself. But now my self-esteem is really rising, and I am grateful to be here.

There are a lot of gay men who feel like, "Well, I'm gonna get it anyway, so why bother?" And I, for the first time in my life, have experienced that. Feeling like, "Oh, I'm a gay man now, in San Francisco. Of course I'm gonna get it." I think it would be really helpful for us to have groups where we can go and sit and talk about this, or just be able to say, "Well, I feel like this."

They invited me to several support groups, but there's the language barrier. There are a lot more in English. Why not Spanish? Why don't they ask us? Why isn't there a Latina group?

Culturally Appropriate Prevention Materials

Participants stated that HIV education, media, and referral materials were developed for nontransgendered populations and the information is not factually or culturally appropriate for the transgender community. For example, MTF individuals are often given HIV education materials that were developed for either women or gay men. However, such materials are usually ineffective because MTFs cannot identify with messages and images that do not fit their bodies or self-images. Both MTF and FTM participants discussed the importance of seeing transgender images that they can identify with in HIV prevention media and education campaigns. There was also a lot of discussion about the need for transgender-specific materials in languages other than English.

My friend and I have never been exposed to any AIDS prevention. It's already a day late and a dollar short for transgenders. Gays don't think of us as gay, we don't think of ourselves as gay, so we ignore half of the advertising that's out there; it doesn't apply.

You always see AIDS posters with two women together or two men together, or a man and a woman, but you never see another transgender person with another man, or woman, or another transgender person.

Unmet Need: HIV Health Services

Primary Health Care for HIV-Positive Transgendered Individuals

By far, the most common area of unmet service need for HIV-infected transgendered people was primary medical care. Many comments were made about physicians' lack of knowledge about the effects and potential dangers of taking hormones and seeking sexual reassignment surgery for those who are living with HIV. HIV-positive participants stated that they receive extremely confusing messages from medical providers and that they need more information about hormone therapy and sexual reassignment surgery to make more informed decisions.

Discussion of the need for improved general health services for people living with HIV centered on the need for affordable, accessible, and transgender-friendly health care and greater inclusion of transgendered persons in AIDS clinical trials.

A lot of doctors discourage transgenders who are HIV positive to go through sex reassignment surgery because it would suppress the immune system. I personally see getting hormones and getting stuck, and I'm not really going anywhere. I feel like I'm in limbo, taking hormone therapy and not able to have the operation. It's affecting my self-esteem and the way I see myself. I think a stronger self-esteem would be a better way to cope with the virus.

I asked my doctor if I could keep using hormones after I found out I was HIV positive, and he told me yes, but then I heard from another source that they can make you ill.

Clinical trials for HIV-infected people—very few, if any, include transgender persons.

I would like to see a health program open that is specific to the needs of the transgender population. I would like for that agency to be culturally sensitive.

HIV Peer Support Groups

Focus group participants discussed the lack of support groups for HIV-infected transgendered individuals to talk about the social, medical, and mental health issues they face. Participants underscored the value of support groups in improving self-esteem, increasing access to health care, and encouraging healthy lifestyles.

> I believe that most of the transgenders that are HIV positive need an outlet, such as support groups.

> There are hundreds of support groups in the city, but there isn't a FTM HIV support group. I've heard things here today that I identify with, that I've never heard before. That says how little is available to us.

Client Advocacy/Case Management

Client advocacy and case management were two important areas of unmet need for transgendered people living with HIV. Participants who were HIV infected stated that they needed client advocacy services such as benefits counseling, legal assistance, and housing placement. The lack of case management services for HIV-infected incarcerated individuals who are released from jail was of concern to participants. Participants related that most transgendered people are able to get adequate medical care when incarcerated, but they are unable to maintain this level of health care once they return to the community.

> If I'm sick and the clinic is all full, I have to go across town . . . and if I don't have bus tokens, I'll have to crawl there, and you have to have below 200 Tcells to get SSI [Supplemental Security Income] . . .being on GA [General Assistance] is not hacking it, you'll live in a fleabag hotel . . . if you want to change your life you've got to change your medical situation.

> A lot of my transgender girlfriends here in jail are HIV positive; the care they receive here is adequate enough, but a majority of them have no resources when they hit the streets to maintain this care, and they go straight down the tubes again, as far as their health, their weight, their taking care of themselves.

I've spent two years waiting for my housing, and now my number is two thousand four, so I don't believe that the HIV housing list moves, and I'm never going to get housing. We need assistance.

I walked into this town with my SSI case, and when I got told on the phone that this clinic had their own lawyer, or had access to one, when I got there, I just got dumped!

Suggestions for Improving Services

Peer Approach to Service Provision

Implementing a peer-based approach to service delivery was thought to be one of the most efficient and effective ways to improve prevention and health care services for the transgendered population. Participants believed that hiring and training MTF and FTM transgendered individuals as support group facilitators, client advocates, substance abuse counselors, media campaign coordinators, case managers, and outreach workers could facilitate access to services for the transgender community. Employing transgendered staff would also provide jobs to a community that has suffered severe employment discrimination.

When I see all these agencies who are being funded all this money to do transgender prevention and provide transgender services, I really find it hard, when I see that some of these agencies are funded to hire four and five outreach workers. And they hire all these outreach workers, and not one of them is transgender.

I've had clients come from an agency, and they're talking about the staff calling them "boy" and "he," and asking them questions, like why they want to do that. If they're going to be serving transgender persons, they should be obligated to make sure that their staff is trained on transgender sensitivity issues, and that their staff is transgender.

We're transgendered men. We might fall into other categories, but there's nothing that's being directed at us. When I hear that an agency is transgender friendly, it sometimes means that there's no transgenders on staff. The book's gotta be written, with us as the subject.

Service Provider Training

The need for transgender sensitivity training for health and social service providers was discussed frequently. Most participants believed that existing providers would not be able to meet the unique needs of this community without more training. The development of guidelines for service provision (particularly for HIV-positive individuals who want to pursue hormone therapy and sexual reassignment surgery) is a critical component of such training efforts. A training unit responsible for developing and implementing in-service trainings should be formed to ensure that systematic training of all service providers takes place on an ongoing basis.

> We're an abomination to society, to the medical and health community. Medical and mental health services are not educated about transgender people. If they're not educated, how can the community get educated from them?

> Make mandatory sensitivity trainings to all service agencies that come in contact with transgender clients.

DISCUSSION OF FINDINGS

To our knowledge, this is the first study to examine qualitatively the HIV risk behaviors and service needs of a large and diverse sample of male-to-female and female-to-male transgendered individuals. The potential for HIV transmission among transgendered individuals and those in their sexual and drug use networks is great. We found alarmingly high levels of HIV risk behaviors, including sex work, injection drug use, and unprotected sex. We also found that many transgendered persons had multiple barriers to accessing needed HIV prevention and health services.

Economic necessity, as a result of severe employment and housing discrimination, results in a reliance on sex work to secure food, shelter, and money for many MTF individuals. Our findings support previous research that has identified a cyclical pattern of sex work and drug use that is difficult to break.[5,8] Once involved in sex work, high rates of drug use and sexual risk taking with multiple partners place this vulnerable population at risk for HIV infection.[1]

Transgendered MTF and FTM populations who do not engage in sex work also appear to be at risk for acquiring HIV. Our findings confirm other qualitative work which found that injection and noninjection drug use is very common, and that many transgendered individuals engage in unprotected sex because it makes them feel sexually validated and increases their self-esteem.[4,5,8] This form of self-validation was particularly important for FTMs who identified as gay or bisexual and had sex with gay men, a troubling finding given the high HIV seroprevalence in San Francisco's gay male population.

Although the need for HIV prevention and health services is great, many transgendered individuals do not access services because of fear of discrimination and dissatisfaction with the quality of care. Focus group participants who had a negative experience trying to access services said they were reluctant to try to obtain services again.

LIMITATIONS AND CONCLUSIONS

Focus groups introduce some limitations that should be acknowledged. The nonprobability sampling methods and qualitative nature of the data compromise our ability to estimate the prevalence of HIV risk behaviors and generalize our findings to transgendered persons in San Francisco. Since only two groups were conducted in a language other than English (the Spanish-speaking groups) and only one FTM-specific group was held, the issues of transgendered persons who speak other languages and FTM individuals may not be adequately captured in this report. Additionally, the study population was largely composed of individuals who have some access to services, since all of the focus groups were conducted at agencies providing HIV prevention or care; our results may fail to represent transgendered persons who are not accessing services.

Despite the aforementioned limitations, our research provides an in-depth description of the HIV risk behaviors and service needs of a large and diverse sample of MTF and FTM individuals. The high levels of unemployment, substance abuse, and homelessness in this population suggest that HIV prevention and health services need to be complemented with job training, education, drug treatment, and housing placement to be effective. Hiring transgendered persons to be involved in the development and implementation of such programs is probably the best way to reach and retain individuals who are most in need of services. To overcome barriers to seeking care and to improve the quality of care delivered, transgender sensitivity training for service providers is also needed. Strengthening prevention and health services for the transgender community is critical to preventing further HIV transmission and facilitating improved health for this high-risk and underserved population.

NOTES

1. Elifson, K.W., Boles, J., Posey, E., Sweat, M., Darrow, W., and Elsea, W. (1993). Male Transvestite Prostitutes and HIV Risk. *American Journal of Public Health* 83(2):260-262.

2. Elifson, K. Boles, J., Sweat, M., Darrow, W., Elsea, W., Green, R. (1989). Seroprevalence of Human Immunodeficiency Virus Among Male Prostitutes. *New England Journal of Medicine* 321:832-833.

3. Peterson, J., Zevin, B., Brody, B. (1996). Characteristics of Transgender Persons Attending a Public Clinic. *Abstracts of the Annual Conference of the American Public Health Association* p. 374.

4. Bockting, W.O., Robinson, E., and Rosser, B.R.S. (1998). Transgender HIV Prevention: A Qualitative Needs Assessment. *AIDS Care* 10(4):505-526.

5. Mason, T.H., Connors, M.M., Kammerer, C.A. (1995). *Transgenders and HIV Risks: Needs Assessment.* Prepared for the Massachusetts Department of Public Health, HIV/AIDS Bureau. Boston: Gender Identity Support Services for Transgenders (GISST).

6. Sandoval, C. (1995). *Focus Group Findings on Transgendered Persons in California.* San Francisco: Polaris Research and Development Inc.

7. Support Center for Nonprofit Management (1994). *Results from a Transgender Focus Group.* San Francisco: Support Center for Nonprofit Management. Prepared for the San Francisco Prevention Planning Council.

8. Yep, G.A., and Pietri, M.P. (1996). *Communicating to the Gender Transposed About HIV/AIDS: An Application of the PRECEDE Framework.* Presented at the 82nd Annual Meeting of the Speech Communication Association, San Diego, California.

Chapter 6

HIV/AIDS and Female-to-Male Transsexuals and Transvestites: Results from a Needs Assessment in Quebec

Viviane K. Namaste

INTRODUCTION

In recent years, public health and epidemiological researchers have focused some attention on transgendered people with respect to HIV/AIDS.[1] The available research, however, generally limits itself to male-to-female (MTF) transsexual and transgendered people, especially those individuals who work as prostitutes. The unique needs of female-to-male (FTM) transsexuals and transvestites are neglected within the existing literature.[2] This chapter reports on some of the preliminary results of the particular needs of FTM people (transsexual, transvestite, and/or transgendered)[3] with regard to HIV/AIDS, drawn from individual interviews conducted with five FTM individuals in Quebec, as well as a discussion group on this topic with FTM individuals at an FTM conference, The Hero's Journey, held in Boston in August 1997. The research yields five major conclusions: (1) there is a lack of informational and educational materials about

I would like to thank several individuals for assistance in gathering and interpreting these data, notably, Henry Rubin, Doug Hein, Ben Singer, Matt Rice, and Dale Altrows.

HIV/AIDS, particularly in reference to FTM identities, sexual practices, and bodies; (2) many FTMs do not consider themselves at risk for HIV/AIDS; (3) a social, administrative, and political context of health care creates conditions wherein FTMs are vulnerable to HIV/AIDS, as evidenced in a lack of access to intramuscular needles (used for the injection of hormones) within needle exchange programs; (4) issues of self-esteem may prevent individuals from adopting low-risk behaviors with respect to the transmission of HIV; and (5) the administrative context of health care and social service delivery excludes FTM transsexuals and transvestites.

BACKGROUND OF THE PROJECT

This research is part of a provincial needs assessment of transsexuals and transvestites in relation to HIV/AIDS in Quebec. Funded by the Centre Quebecois de Coordination sur le SIDA, a provincial government coordinating body, the project sought to identify the primary needs of transsexuals and transvestites in relation to HIV/AIDS within the province of Quebec. The needs assessment targeted three cities in Quebec: Montreal, Quebec City, and Hull. The research was institutionally located in the community organization CACTUS, *Centre d'action auprès des toxicomanes utilisateurs de seringues,* a needle exchange located in downtown Montreal. A transsexual outreach worker employed by CACTUS identified the need for such a project and coordinated the efforts of transsexuals and tranvestites, researchers, public health representatives, as well as provincial and federal health officials to begin to address this issue. A community-based advisory committee, with a majority of transsexual/transvestite members, supervised the research in the development, implementation, and interpretation of the results.

This needs assessment particularly focused on how transsexuals and transvestites relate to and experience health care and social services. Building on the existing research literature of marginalized populations such as prostitutes and drug users, the project situated HIV within a global context of health care. Within such a paradigm, it is argued that members of marginalized populations must fulfill their primary health care and social service needs first; they can integrate low HIV risk behaviors only after their more immediate needs have been met.[4] Quebec's national policy with respect to HIV adopts this orientation.[5]

Whereas the existing literature on HIV and transgendered people is primarily limited to an epidemiological and/or public health perspective, this research project offers a sociological investigation of the problem. Thus, rather than focusing exclusively on individual behaviors, the research examines the social, political, and economic factors which marginalize transsexuals and transvestites in Quebec and which may place these individuals at increased risk of HIV transmission. A review of the XI International AIDS Conference in Vancouver makes clear the importance of such a focus:

> Although some efforts beyond the provision of information and the targeting of individual decision-making were described, there continues to be a great deal of interest, particularly shown in media attention during the conference, on the psychological and individual factors determining "risk," rather than social and economic factors that create conditions for "vulnerability."[6]

The needs assessment aims to offer precisely such a sociological explanation of social, economic, and political factors that create conditions of vulnerability to HIV for transsexuals and transvestites in Quebec. This chapter reports on the results explicitly concerned with FTMs; a more general overview of transsexual/transvestite health care in Quebec is available in the final report of the project.[7]

METHODS

In recent years, public health research has recognized the value of qualitative research methods, particularly with respect to marginalized populations. While an epidemiological framework can offer important data on the prevalence of particular diseases within a population, the reasons for the transmission of such diseases, either within a population or outside of it, are not always evident from aggregate statistical data.[8] Qualitative research can play a useful role in this regard, both in furthering our understanding of how diseases are conceptualized and experienced, and in the evaluation of community-based programs.

The needs assessment identified several topics for investigation: hormone therapy, gender identity clinics, addictions, prisons, ethnocultural minorities, HIV/AIDS, FTMs, and civil status.[9] The data were gathered in two ways: (1) through individual interviews with five FTM transsexuals or tranvestites in Quebec, and (2) through a discussion group with FTMs, researchers, social workers, and health care professionals at an FTM conference in Boston, held in August 1997. Although the American location of this conference is outside the terms of the needs assessment, the data are nonetheless worthy of consideration, given the dearth of research on the topic of FTMs and HIV/AIDS. Moreover, such a comparative analysis is further useful since attention to health care within an American context can illuminate the social and administrative organization of health care in Quebec.

In addition to responding to questions posed by an interviewer, or topics introduced by the facilitator of a focus/discussion group, FTMs were involved in the generation, validation, and interpretation of this research. In Quebec, FTMs were represented at the advisory committee, which reviewed and approved the interview guide. Once the initial interviews were completed in Quebec, participants were invited to attend a public session to verify the preliminary results; a session was held in each city of Montreal, Quebec, and Hull.[10] These forums sought to solicit the feedback and comments of participants, and to validate the research results before they were presented to the government in a final report. FTMs who attended the focus/discussion group at the conference in Boston were asked to validate the research by reviewing a written summary of the workshop to be prepared by the researcher; it was promised that any modifications or errors would be corrected, and alternate interpretations of the findings would also be recorded before the research was published. Moreover, as part of a research contract, I agreed to publish a summary of the results in a forum widely accessible to American FTMs, such as *The FTM Newsletter* or the American transsexual magazine *Transsexual News Telegraph.*

Although time-consuming and labor-intensive, the process of generating, collecting, interpreting, and verifying the data was aimed at transforming the relations FTMs have with health care and social services, by giving them an opportunity to formulate their own research questions, identify their own needs, and offer their own interpretations.[11] In this regard, I hoped to include FTMs in the research process as active subjects, rather than as mere objects of inquiry. Such a strategy attempts to forge collaborative relations between researchers and members of marginalized communities, relations that have immediate and practical relevance in the development, implementation, and evaluation of community-based programs that may emerge as a result of the research.[12]

RESULTS

The needs assessment indicates five salient issues with regard to FTMs and HIV/AIDS. These five issues constitute a global situation in which FTMs are at risk for HIV/AIDS and suggest some useful directions for the development of community-based programs.

First, there is a lack of informational and educational materials about FTM bodies, sexualities, and identities. For instance, participants in the discussion group stated that, although it is known that some FTMs enjoy and practice vaginal sex, little is known about the risk factors involved: Do male hormones dry out the vagina of an FTM transsexual, thus requiring that any FTM who has penile-vaginal intercourse use a latex condom, as well as a water-based lubricant?

Second, FTMs do not consider themselves to be at risk for HIV. This finding was especially remarkable in the individual interviews conducted in Quebec: participants often commented that HIV affected street people, intravenous drug users, and/or prostitutes.[13] The absence of a penis and/or semen in FTMs was cited as one reason why FTMs are not at risk for HIV.[14]

A third finding relates to the social and political context of health care for FTMs, most particularly, the availability of intramuscular needles for the injection of hormones. Participants at the conference in Boston claimed that access to these needles remains difficult in the United States, since the possession or use of drugs is criminalized. Moreover, FTMs reported that many individuals use two needles to inject—a large gauge needle to withdraw the fluid from its container (it is immersed in oil and quite thick) and a smaller needle to actually inject the hormones into the body. If access to sterile syringes is an issue in the first place, then the risk of HIV transmission, hepatitis, and/or other health complications increases with the number of needles used for each injection. Intramuscular hormone needles are available through some needle exchange programs in the United States, although FTMs maintained that they often face tremendous difficulties in accessing them. In San Francisco, for instance, intramuscular needles are only available through a site for women (including male-to-female transsexuals).[15] Although this program will bring intramuscular needles to another site for FTMs or other men (such as those who use steroids), such arrangements need to be made in advance. As such, in practical terms, there is a poor availability of intramuscular needles for FTMs in San Francisco. Access to hormones themselves was also raised as an issue by participants at the FTM conference. It was reported that FTMs who live near the Mexican border can buy hormones without a prescription in Mexico and transport them across the border into the United States. This strategy, however, raises the problem of potential legal difficulties upon entering the United States, since the transportation of hormones without a prescription can be considered trafficking of contraband drugs across national borders. Furthermore, it does not necessarily resolve the issue of access to intramuscular needles.

The information presented by Quebec interviewees contrasts sharply with the data generated at the conference in Boston. Intramuscular needles are readily available through some needle exchange programs, notably, CACTUS in Montreal. These needles (as well as intravenous needles) can also be purchased at the pharmacy. FTM transsexuals in Quebec can obtain sterile needles for injection—even needles of different gauges, should they so desire. In this light, the sociopolitical context of health care is an important and immediate determinant of health. The criminilization and repression of (intravenous) drug use creates conditions of vulnerability to HIV. As other research has demonstrated, a lack of access to sterile syringes in a particular jurisdiction correlates to increased seropositive rates in the population of that region.[16]

A fourth finding of the needs assessment focuses on the issue of self-esteem. FTM participants at the discussion group stated that FTMs experience difficulties in finding sexual partners. Given such difficulties, FTMs may not protect themselves and/or their sexual partners during sexual intercourse for fear of rejection. FTMs who identified as gay and/or bisexual men stated that some FTMs only offer oral sex to other men, so as not to compromise their own transsexual status. Ridicule, harassment, physical violence, and sexual assault upon discovery or disclosure of one's transgendered status were cited as reasons individuals would not disclose their transgendered status. FTMs also remarked that some of them have "no touching" zones on the body: a criterion to which many gay men are not accustomed in their sexual relations. Other FTMs said that they enjoyed penile-vaginal intercourse, but that they could not broach this subject within a gay male context such as a support group.

Finally, interviewees and participants of the discussion group at the FTM conference contended that the administration of social services excludes transsexuals and transvestites. FTMs can be (and are often) classified as women in the daily practices of different administrative agencies. Gender-exclusive forms or counseling practices are different examples of how transgendered people must categorize themselves as "men" or "women" and thus deny the complexity of their bodies, identities, and histories.

CONCLUSION

In addition to documenting the needs identified by FTMs with respect to HIV/AIDS, the results of the needs assessment suggest some useful orientations for program and service delivery, as well as some significant reflections on the import of qualitative research methods.

Given that many FTMs do not consider themselves to be at risk for HIV/AIDS, community-based programs and services ought not to emphasize HIV/AIDS in their delivery but, rather, integrate HIV/AIDS education subtly into a more global program of health care information and services. An approach that focuses on health promotion would attract a larger (and probably more diverse) audience of FTMs than one that is marketed through the theme of HIV.[17]

The results also demonstrate that the sociopolitical context of health care creates conditions of vulnerability to HIV. For instance, in regions where availability of intravenous needles is poor, the population often shows a higher seroprevalence rate. This study extends this line of thought to a transgendered population: in jurisdictions where intramuscular needles are not easily obtainable, transsexuals are at increased risk for HIV. How health is understood politically translates directly into how health services are administered, which in turn impacts on how and why people are at risk for HIV.

Finally, the study illustrates the value of qualitative research methods in such an inquiry. The nature of the knowledge collected within this needs assessment could not be gathered through statistical, quantitative methods. Qualitative methods thus lend themselves well to research with marginalized populations, or populations about whom little is known. Furthermore, the very process of research can help forge collaborative relations between researchers and their subjects—a collaboration that can facilitate the social integration of these individuals. In allowing marginalized individuals to ask their own questions, identify their own needs, and validate their own research, qualitative research benefits the scholarly community of scientists and researchers as well as the members of the population under investigation. As such, qualitative research methods can play an important role in a broader process of community development.

NOTES

1. James Inciardi and Hilary Surratt (1992). "Male transvestite workers and HIV in Rio de Janeiro, Brazil," *Journal of Drug Issues* 27(1): 135-146; P. Gattari, L. Spizzichino, C. Valenzi, M. Zaccarelli, and G. Reeza (1992). "Behavioural patterns and HIV infection among drug using transvestites practising prostitution in Rome," *AIDS Care* 4(1): 83-87; Theresa Mason, Margaret Connors, and Cornelia Kammerer (1995). *Transgenders and HIV Risks: Needs Assessment* (Boston: Massachusetts Department of Public Health); W.O. Bockting, B.E. Robinson, and B.R.S. Rosser (1998). "Transgender HIV prevention: A qualitative needs assessment," *AIDS Care* 10(4): 505-526.

2. An innovative program on HIV/AIDS for FTMs was conceived and developed in Boston, however. See Doug Hein and Michael Kirk (Boston Public Health AIDS Services) (1997). "Education and soul-searching: The Enterprise HIV Prevention Group," presentation at Hero's Journey Conference, Boston, Massachusetts. August. This report appears also as Chapter 7 in this book.

3. In French, the term "gender" does not exist, nor does its corollary, "transgender." Since my research is based on the experiences of people in Quebec, a French-speaking jurisdiction, I will not refer to an umbrella category of *transgendered people* but rather to *transsexuals* and *transvestites*. This terminological choice is not to deny the existence of individuals who live in a gender other than that assigned to them at birth, and who may take hormones and/or have certain surgeries, yet who do not (in English) call themselves transsexual. It is, rather, to begin with the terminological categories employed by the francophone participants of this research project.

4. For a useful overview of different research studies and program evaluations that draw this conclusion, see Purnima Mane, Peter Aggleton, Gary Dowsett, Richard Parker, Geeta Rao Gupta, Sandra Anderson, Stefano Bertozzi, Eric Chevalier, Martina Clark, Noerine Kaleeba, et al. (1996). "Summary of Track D: Social science: Research, policy and action," *AIDS* 10 (suppl. 3): S123-S132.

5. Ministère de la sante et des services sociaux, Direction generale de la sante publique, *Strategie quebecoise de lutte contre le sida. Phase 4 orientations 1997-2002* (Quebec: Gouvernement du Quebec, 1997).

6. Purnima Mane, Peter Aggleton, Gary Dowsett, Richard Parker, Geeta Rao Gupta, Sandra Anderson, Stefano Bertozzi, Eric Chevalier, Martina Clark, Noerine Kaleeba, et al. (1996). "Summary of Track D: Social science: Research, policy and action," *AIDS* 10 (suppl. 3): S127.

7. Viviane K. Namaste (1998). *Évaluation des besoins: Les travesti(e)s et les transsexuel(le)s au Quebec à l'égard du VIH/sida* (Montreal: Report submitted to the Centre Quebecois de Coordination sur le SIDA, May 1998). Due to space limitations, this chapter does not present some very important data with respect to the change of name and the change of sex for FTMs in Quebec, and how these administrative procedures marginalize FTMs and make them vulnerable to the transmission of HIV. Readers are invited to consult the final report cited here for an in-depth discussion of this question.

8. Ministère de la sante et des services sociaux, Direction generale de la sante publique, *Strategie quebecoise de lutte contre le sida. Phase 4 orientations 1997-2002* (Quebec: Gouvernement du Quebec, 1997).

9. These substantive areas of inquiry were identified by the advisory committee of the project.

10. All of the FTM participants, however, lived in the Montreal region.

11. See Benoît Gauthier (1992). "La recherche-action." In Benoît Gauthier, ed. *Recherche sociale: De la problematique à la collecte des donnees* (Sillery, Quebec: Presses de l'Universite du Quebec): 517-533.

12. See Henri Lamoureux, Robert Mayer, and Jean Panet-Raymond (1984). *L'Intervention communautaire* (Montreal: Éditions Saint-Martin).

13. A methodological question must be posed at this point. Since the discussion group at the conference was clearly labeled as one pertaining to HIV/AIDS, it would only attract FTMs interested in addressing this subject. Thus, it is not that FTMs in Quebec do not consider themselves to be at risk for HIV while those in the United States do.

14. Field notes, September 12, 1997.

15. Personal correspondence with Matt Rice, October 14, 1997.

16. Alex Wodak and Peter Lurie (1996). "A Tale of two countries: Attempts to control HIV among injecting drug users in Australia and the United States," *Journal of Drug Issues* 27(1): 117-134.

17. A more in-depth discussion of valuable orientation of services for transsexuals and transvestites is available in Viviane K. Namaste (1998). *Évaluation des besoins: Les travesti(e)s et les transsexuel(le)s à l'égard du VIH/sida* (Montreal: Report submitted to the Centre Quebecois de Coordination sur le SIDA.)

Chapter 7

Education and Soul-Searching: The Enterprise HIV Prevention Group

Douglas Hein
Michael Kirk

INTRODUCTION

The prevention group, Education and Soul-Searching, is adapted from a curriculum developed for HIV-negative gay and bisexual men by the Boston Public Health Commission and the Fenway Community Health Center in 1994. Although the structure of the Enterprise workshops is based on the 1994 intervention, the issues addressed in workshop sessions are determined by female-to-male (FTM) participants. The workshops include education, discussion, and participatory exercises focused on (1) HIV/STD transmission and risk reduction information, (2) testosterone therapy and its impact on sexual behavior, (3) social and cultural issues that marginalize FTMs and affect their risk for infection, (4) disclosure of transsexual identity to sexual partners, (5) coping with gender-discordant strategies for managing behavioral risk, (6) developing language that accurately describes sexual desire and intention, (7) understanding the role of sexual pleasure and its connection to FTM identity, (8) using risk

The authors would like to thank Buck, Mykael Hawley, and all the men who participated in Education and Soul-Searching. Their honesty and "courageous hearts" made the prevention workshops possible. Correspondence and requests for materials can be sent to Douglas Hein at <doug_hein@ bphc.org>.

management strategies that focus on the values and meanings of risk behaviors; and (9) forming connections with people outside the FTM community as allies, sexual partners, and significant others.

This chapter will focus briefly on Enterprise's membership, mission, and history as well as recent paradigm shifts in HIV prevention. The workshop sessions will be described fully.

A BRIEF HISTORY OF ENTERPRISE

Enterprise, founded by members of the FTM community in Greater Boston, functioned as a peer support group for transsexual men from 1993 to 1998. The group met weekly and provided a supportive environment for members to socialize, mentor one another, address medical issues related to hormonal therapy and surgery, and offer emotional support. Enterprise members reported many of the same difficulties as FTMs from other parts of the United States: (1) fear of lack of access to competent medical care and social services,[1] (2) fears about disclosure of one's transsexual status, (3) social marginalization, and (4) fears regarding physical violence.

Enterprise also provided opportunities for community visibility and individual empowerment. Group members were active locally and nationally in promoting awareness about FTM issues through participation in educational forums, conferences, art exhibitions, and performances. In 1997, Enterprise sponsored four events in Greater Boston that significantly increased the organization's visibility. A few hundred people attended an evening of music and celebration in late March to commemorate the publication of Loren Cameron's book *Body Alchemy: Transsexual Portraits.*[2] In early April, the New England Film Festival premiered *You Don't Know Dick: Courageous Hearts of Transsexual Men*[3] and named the film Best Documentary of 1996. In June, Enterprise cosponsored the first FTM contingent for Boston Gay Pride. In August, Enterprise shared sponsorship of The Hero's Journey: The Third Annual FTM Conference of the Americas with two other FTM groups, the Officer's Club and the local chapter of American Boyz.

From 1993 to 1996, Enterprise members met weekly in one another's homes. During 1996, the membership used a community room in Boston for meetings. From 1997 to 1998, Enterprise meetings were held in Waltham, Massachusetts, at the International Foundation for Gender Education (IFGE), an organization focused on support and advocacy for the MTF/FTM transgender/transsexual community. In 1999, a founding member of Enterprise established the FTM Center in collaboration with the Boston Medical Center. This peer-level support group meets bimonthly for FTMs who are undergoing or have completed their transition.

PARADIGM SHIFTS IN HIV PREVENTION

In 1991, HIV test sites in Boston began to see more gay men engaging in repeat or routine testing.[4] HIV counseling staff realized that concerns about HIV were affecting their clients' quality of life, and some men seemed to be experiencing difficulty in sustaining safer-sex practices.[5] Mental health clinicians treating gay and bisexual men began to publish articles citing the psychological effects of ten years of behavioral vigilance and personal loss. Psychotherapists reported patients with AIDS-related depression, anxiety, hypochondria, impotence, survivor guilt, sexual anorexia (avoidance of sex), alcoholism, and drug use.[6]

Research and popular journalism about HIV prevention between 1991 and 1995 focused on four areas of concern: (1) many uninfected gay men were survivors of trauma and loss; (2) HIV-negative gay men experienced confusion about generalized prevention messages that failed to differentiate between the needs of infected and uninfected men; (3) HIV prevention strategies employed during the first ten years of the epidemic were information based and did not seem to help men sustain behavior change over time; and (4) prevention strategies based on harm reduction and risk management were designed to promote sustained behavior change by addressing the cultural meanings of risk behaviors in specific populations.[7]

The Boston Public Health Commission and the Fenway Community Health Center began a three-week support and education group for uninfected gay men in 1994.[8] The group model was designed to extend HIV-negative posttest counseling for men at risk and was based on an existing support and education group for HIV-positive individuals in Boston.[9] The HIV-negative support and education group continues to meet monthly at the Fenway Community Health Center.

Although the 1994 intervention targets uninfected gay men, project staff developed the model with the intention that it be replicated for other populations at risk. Group members contribute significantly to the content of each session, prioritize issues they want to address, and develop prevention strategies based on their particular needs.

In the process of planning an HIV prevention group for FTMs, we realized that some of their concerns and experiences were similar to the concerns of gay men in 1991: (1) many FTM transsexuals experience both loss and renewal as they transition toward living fully as men; (2) HIV prevention education based on gender and sexual orientation does not address the specific needs of FTMs; (3) information-based prevention strategies do not address the complexity of transsexual bodies, cultures, and sexual relationships,[10] and (4) harm reduction and risk management strategies can be used to address the specific health concerns and sexual practices of FTM transsexuals.

THE ENTERPRISE PREVENTION WORKSHOPS

The authors met through a local AIDS services organization in 1995. They agreed that most HIV prevention programming in Boston for transgenders and transsexuals focused on the needs of the MTF community, and that FTMs needed programs focused on their particular risks. Periodically for the next two years, the authors offered to conduct an HIV prevention group at Enterprise. Enterprise members responded with ambivalence; HIV did not seem to be a priority in their lives during this time. In 1997, the membership decided that they wanted a series of prevention workshops, and Education and Soul-Searching[11] was promoted through a mailing by an Enterprise member.

The two-year time period is mentioned because it seems to correlate with some of the issues discussed later by men in the prevention workshops. The authors discussed four possible reasons for the men's ambivalence: (1) members found it difficult to trust someone from outside the group, especially a non-FTM facilitator associated with health care; (2) they were focused on their gender transition and needed to devote their time, energy, and resources to helping one another manage those changes; (3) HIV was one of many health issues that concerned and marginalized them; and (4) dealing with HIV meant facing their fears about infection.

Two series of workshops were conducted in 1997 and 1998. Each series consisted of three sessions that spanned a two-month period, with a one-, two-, or three-week interval between each session.

Scheduling was based on the needs and time constraints of Enterprise members. Each session was approximately two hours long.

The first series of workshops was held in Boston during the winter of 1997. The second series was held in Waltham during the spring of 1998. Four to six men attended each workshop session, and all identified as FTM transsexuals. Although heterosexual, bisexual, and gay men attended the workshops, most of the participants identified as gay or bisexual. Heterosexual men were more likely to drop out before the third session.

Participants were in different stages of gender transition. Some had been taking testosterone for years, had undergone multiple surgeries, and were living fully as men. Other participants were just starting their transition, taking low doses of testosterone, and contemplating surgical options.

For purposes of coherence and clarity, we will combine content from both the 1997 and 1998 series of workshops in our descriptions of workshop components. The descriptions of sessions imply that topics were discussed sequentially in a predetermined order. In reality, group discussions were loosely organized around the multiple themes addressed in this chapter. Each workshop was facilitated by a non-FTM HIV prevention counselor and a peer facilitator from Enterprise.

During the first workshop session, facilitators employed simple ground rules, asked participants to talk about their reasons for attending the group, and discussed the risks and benefits of participation. They used the beginning and ending of each session as check-in time regarding members' needs and expectations. Participants' discussion responses were written on an easel chart during each session.

Session I

Understanding Social and Cultural Risk Factors

BY YOUR RESPONSE TO DANGER IT IS
EASY TO TELL HOW YOU HAVE LIVED
AND WHAT HAS BEEN DONE TO YOU.
YOU SHOW WHETHER YOU WANT TO STAY ALIVE,
WHETHER YOU THINK YOU DESERVE TO,
AND WHETHER YOU BELIEVE
IT'S ANY GOOD TO ACT.[12]

This epigram is used to initiate discussion about (1) life circumstances that increase personal vulnerability; (2) life circumstances that contribute to personal strength; and (3) the effect of gender transition on one's ability to manage health concerns.

Participants seemed to value the opportunity to talk about themselves as well as their concerns about HIV. Some expressed relief that the workshop offered more than generalized information about safer sex and prescriptive advice about condoms and dental dams.

Building Trust Between FTM Participants and the Facilitator

As stated previously, one of the facilitators was a non-FTM HIV prevention counselor. Although he had discussed FTM issues extensively with the peer facilitator and read most of the existing literature on FTM culture and sexuality, his experience with FTMs from different backgrounds and stages of gender transition was limited.

Part of the first session involved a conscious dialogue between the non-FTM facilitator and participants. This facilitator spoke briefly about what he had learned so far and asked group members to share as much information as they wanted about their lives as transsexual men. Although workshop participants knew one another well, they willingly shared their personal stories with the facilitator. This included information about their jobs, gender histories, current stages of transition, sexual orientation, and the impact of hormones and surgery. They also talked about relationships with co-workers, parents, siblings, significant others, spouses, and children.

Session II

Describing HIV-Testing Experience

Most of the men in the group had been screened for HIV at least once, and some were contemplating retesting in the future. The facilitators asked the men to talk about their testing experiences as well as any other concerns they had related to testing. Participants described the difficulties of dealing with intake forms and health care practices that did not include transgender and/or transsexual as gender categories. Group members also expressed ambivalence about disclosing their transsexual status during pre- and posttest counseling; they valued being perceived as men and found it difficult to trust counseling staff. Facilitators provided information about standards of care for

HIV counseling and testing, and group members described their experiences with testing programs in Boston that specialize in the needs of transsexuals.

Sharing Personal Stories Related to HIV

People talked about their fears and confusion about managing risk for HIV infection. Some participants knew people with HIV; others had marginal contact with the epidemic and limited knowledge about safer sex. People perceived HIV risk in relation to their concerns as transsexuals and identified and discussed the following themes: (1) disclosure of transsexual identity to sexual partners, (2) disclosure of HIV status to sexual partners, (3) talking with sexual partners about testing, (4) coping with gender-discordant strategies for managing risk, and (5) developing sexual language consistent with gender identity.

Educating About HIV/STD Transmission

Participants had specific questions about safer-sex behaviors, and some men needed basic information about the prevention of HIV and STDs. Men expressed concerns about new sexual behaviors, especially ones that correlated with changes in sexual orientation or involved sexual experimentation. This seemed particularly true for participants who were having sex with men, and their questions reflected an increased interest in oral-penile and oral-anal sex.

Talking to Partners About HIV Status and Safer Sex

Participants wanted to talk to sexual partners about HIV status and safer sex. They also asked for strategies that would help them negotiate sexual boundaries. Facilitators helped participants discuss (1) ways to introduce information about HIV early in the encounter or relationship, (2) the risks and benefits to disclosure, (3) the meanings of disclosure for both negative and positive people, (4) the anticipation of one's reactions and responses to partner disclosure, and (5) the establishment of trust with sexual partners.

At first, participants seemed focused on HIV disclosure as a strategy to avoid infection. As group members talked more extensively about the meanings of disclosure for infected and uninfected people, they asked more questions about psychosocial issues for people with HIV.

Some of the men expressed appreciation regarding similarities between coming out as HIV positive and disclosing one's FTM identity.

Participants also began to understand the limitations of disclosure as a prevention strategy, and that in the absence of established trust, negotiating safer sex was an essential part of self-protection.[13] Discussion focused on simple ways to set sexual boundaries (1) introducing HIV risk management as mutually beneficial for both partners, (2) expressing appreciation of a partner's sexual skill, physical attributes, erotic capacity, and/or emotional sensitivity, (3) stating clearly one's boundaries regarding safety, and (4) asking one's partner to assist in identifying mutually pleasurable sexual alternatives.

Participants also discussed nonverbal strategies for sexual risk management. Some men stayed partially clothed during sex to avoid intercourse as well as the disclosure of their transsexual status. Other men used body language to convey sexual boundaries. The facilitators reinforced the effectiveness of using one's body to change power dynamics, avoid unprotected sex, and send signals to partners about sexual alternatives.

Session III

Defining HIV Prevention Strategies

This didactic section defines three different levels of HIV prevention (1) *Risk Reduction* is the informational component of behavior change in which education about HIV transmission and risk reduction supplies, such as condoms and bleach, are provided for people at risk, (2) *Risk Management* is supportive education and counseling that empowers individuals to make decisions about behavior change by considering both risk reduction guidelines and issues related to the social, cultural, and personal meanings of sexual behaviors.[14] (3) *Harm Reduction* is an intermediate intervention especially useful for substance users, in which avoiding infection and injury takes priority over drug treatment and abstinence.[15]

Often the terms risk reduction, risk management, and harm reduction are used interchangeably. In this section, we present these methods as related but fundamentally different prevention practices. Risk reduction promotes behavior change through guidelines provided by an external source. Risk management and harm reduction are client centered, focus on sustaining behavior change over time, and help internalize the process of behavior change by shifting the locus of control back to the individual.

Understanding the Links Between Sex and the Brain

This section provides information about human sexual response and addresses why education about HIV transmission does not always result in successful behavior change.

Education is a cognitive function that happens in the brain cortex. The cortex controls knowledge and awareness and is the learning center of the brain. Sexual behavior is a limbic function that happens in the brain stem. This part of the brain controls one's emotions, behavior, and motivation as well as one's sense of smell and other involuntary actions of the body. Anger, rage, fear, hunger, and satiation are all instinctual responses connected to the brain stem. Sexual response (including penile and clitoral erections, pre-ejaculation, ejaculation, and vaginal lubrication) is an *involuntary* response to stimuli.[16]

The following pairs of words are used to illustrate the differences between cortical and limbic functions. Facilitators asked group members to brainstorm their own lists of comparative responses under the headings *thinking* and *feeling*. This exercise prepares participants for subsequent discussion about the *meanings of behaviors* and the *roles of sexual pleasure*. The goal of this part of the curriculum is to help group members express their motivations and desires for particular sexual behaviors and promote communication between cognitive and limbic states of being.[17]

Brain Cortex		Brain Stem
Cognitive		Limbic
Learning center		Pleasure center
Thinking	*The Meanings of Behaviors*	Feeling
Mind	*The Roles of Pleasure*	Body
Logic		Passion
Reason		Desire
Control		Spontaneous

Participants in one workshop formulated a different interpretation of the previous exercise. These men viewed *thinking* as *risking death* and correlated facts and knowledge about HIV with avoiding infection. They viewed *feeling* as *risking life* and correlated the expression of sexual desire to their survival as new men. These participants considered sexual energy to be as essential to their survival as breathing. They also valued sexual experimentation and desire and regarded sexual feelings as fundamental elements of masculine expression and identity.

Using Risk Management and Harm Reduction

The following table illustrates a preparatory exercise used to help participants express personal values about pleasure and meaning. The use of a sport such as in-line skating is intentional. Usually someone in the group had engaged in the sport, and in-line skating parallels sexual activity in that it can be both hazardous and exhilarating. Participants were asked to brainstorm responses to four headings while one of the facilitators recorded their responses on an easel chart.

Pleasurable Behavior	Meaning of Behavior	What Are the Risks?	Risk Management
In-line Skating	Accomplishment	Falling	Practice
	Being athletic	Injury to self	Protective gear
	Skill	Humiliation	Skating defensively
	Showing off	Embarrassment	Using empty lot
	Youth	Failure	Buddy system
	Speed	Rejection	Lessons
	Control		Level terrain
	Grace		Avoid rush hour
	Elation		Avoid weekends
	Watching men/ women		Knowing how to stop
	Chance to flirt		

After the preparatory exercise, the group participants were asked to choose a sexual behavior for discussion. During the first workshop cycle, all the men who participated in this exercise identified as gay or bisexual. Participants chose to discuss *performing oral sex on a man.* Participants stated that the italicized responses were connected to their identities as FTMs.

Pleasurable Behavior	Meaning of Behavior	What Are the Risks?	Risk Management
Performing oral sex on a man	Arousing Feels good Smell/taste Dick grows hard during act Visual In your face Reciprocal Skill (making him want it/making him cum) Creative (the art of sucking dick) Dominant Cum His body (thighs/ass/balls) *Affirming my maleness* *My identity as a gay man* *Sex with an equal* *Identify with his penis* *Celebrating maleness* *Cock energy* *Nourishment from cum* *Penis as friend* *Powerful for both partners*	HIV STDs Being a receptacle Indifference from partner *Feeling used* *Where will this lead/disclosing gender identity* *Objectifying partner/his dick* *Identify with his cock/then it's over* *Envy* *Grief* *Anger* *Reacting to sexual situations with female social behaviors*	*Working on self-esteem* *Talking to other FTMs/getting support* *Avoiding self-recrimination* *Looking for signs/signals/cues from partner* *Choosing not to disclose gender identity* *Avoiding sexual deprivation* *Learning male social behaviors*

KEY ISSUES FOR WORKSHOP PARTICIPANTS

Education and Soul-Searching provided a structured environment for participants to address the complex relationship between FTM identity and HIV risk management. Group members engaged in frank discussion about their bodies, current sexual relationships, and meaningful sexual behaviors. Themes evolved that require further examination and discourse.

The Roles and Meanings of Sexual Behaviors

Participants attached meaning and value to behaviors that (1) expressed their masculine identities, (2) validated their maleness, (3) celebrated their lives as men, and (4) affirmed their sexual identities and orientations.

For FTMs who identified as gay and bisexual, sexual encounters with biological males provided opportunities to experience gender equality. Gay sex was described as *man to man* and reciprocal for both partners regarding power, control, and submission. Sex with men also allowed participants to develop affinities with their partners' genitals. One group member described viewing his partner's penis as a friend. Other participants experienced vicarious enjoyment of male genitals. Group members also valued sexual intimacy with other men because it provided access to what one participant called *cock energy.* Some participants believed that having male energy was as important to their transition as having a male body. Semen had significant value as a source of male energy and nourishment.[18]

The Emotional Risks of Sexual Behaviors

HIV prevention usually focuses on the physical and health-related risks associated with unprotected sex. Although the facilitators provided factual information about HIV transmission, group members expressed several issues related to the emotional risks they experienced as FTMs (1) fear of disclosing one's transsexual identity during sexual encounters, (2) fluctuating self-esteem related to the incremental nature of gender transition,[19] (3) gender-discordant sexual language and prevention strategies, (4) objectification of male sex partners and their genitals, and (5) envy of their male partners' genitals.

One participant related that simply being *perceived* as a man by potential male or female sexual partners predisposed him to emotional and physical risk. He described the profound validation he continues to feel being recognized as male, and the difficulty of asserting his needs when his gender identity is at stake; doing so might jeopardize his acceptability as a sexual partner, complicate the encounter, and end in rejection.

Other participants described sexual encounters in which they chose not to disclose their transsexual status. This usually involved staying partially or fully dressed during sexual acts. One man recounted keeping his briefs on during an encounter and gaining sexual pleasure by rubbing against his partner's body. Other participants reported feeling frustrated by sexual experiences focused primarily on their partners' pleasure. Although group members enjoyed performing oral sex and masturbation on other men, their needs for attention and release were sometimes deferred or ignored.

Participants talked about the incremental nature of their gender transitions and its effect on self-confidence in sexual situations. Some men stated that their sexual self-esteem fluctuated, and that variations in sexual confidence seemed linked to concerns about ambiguous gender presentation. They were not interested in *passing* as men; they wanted to *be* men and sometimes felt understandably at odds with the incremental nature of gender transition.

One participant reported being at risk for HIV early in his transition. He described responding to sexual situations with passivity and thought that this reflected his years of being socialized as female. This man told the group that acquiring male social behaviors was one of his strategies for managing risk; acting male equated with being male, and he felt more confident with both male and female partners in asserting his needs.

Group members struggled with gender-discordant language when describing sexual situations. Most group members were living fully as men, and many had undergone testosterone therapy, chest surgeries, and hysterectomies. None of the participants had completed genital reconstruction. Group members described sexual experiences in ways that felt consistent with their socialization as new men. Participants referred to some sexual acts as *fucking* and acknowledged that actual penetration was limited. They referred to masturbation as *jerking off* and to their genitals as *cocks* or *dicks,* with the recognition that their choices regarding genital reconstruction were yet to be resolved.[20]

Group members valued condoms because they provided male-identified options for safer intercourse and oral sex but found them difficult or impossible to use. When one group member related his struggles with safer sex, other participants raised the possibility of adapting dental dams for different sexual acts. He shuddered as he told the group that he associated dental dams with vaginal sex and being female; they were not an option, even if it meant contracting HIV.

Dealing with Grief and Loss

Participants agreed that sexual intimacy created opportunities to express their maleness, experiment with new behaviors, and achieve gender authenticity. Group members also described the challenges they sometimes experienced when having sex with other men. Some participants envied their partner's genitals and felt anger and resentment about the adjustments and compromises that FTMs are often forced to make regarding genital reconstruction. Sex with men also seemed to reawaken existential conflicts for group members. They experienced moments when they continued to feel cheated by nature, disappointed by their bodies, and unfairly limited regarding sexual function and pleasure.[21]

CONCLUSION

This chapter documented an HIV prevention program for FTM transsexuals. The purpose of the intervention was to help participants manage HIV in healthy ways. Implicit in that goal is the value of staying uninfected. Group members were encouraged to define health in their own terms, and for most men, remaining HIV negative was a primary goal. They seemed to perceive HIV as synonymous with stigma and loss, and being HIV positive was considered *one more strike in addition to being FTM.*

The content of workshop sessions focused as much on sexual health as HIV prevention. Participants valued the opportunity to talk about transsexual health, sexual orientation, and human sexual response.

One unstated goal of Education and Soul-Searching was eventual peer leadership of a prevention project based on the intervention. Transsexual professionals and peers have been essential in the provision of culturally competent HIV prevention both nationally and internationally. However, using a non-FTM facilitator had value for group members. Although he needed additional information from group members about their lives, he was knowledgeable about FTM culture. He understood issues related to sexual orientation, had years of experience in HIV prevention, and wanted to advocate for transsexual health services. Some participants viewed him as a male role model; others saw him as a community ally worthy of trust.

This intervention has not been evaluated regarding program efficacy and prospective outcomes for group members. However, the 1994 prevention project for uninfected gay men has been qualitatively evaluated.[22] This chapter examines how theories of life stress, cognitive escape, social learning, psychoeducation, and social networks inform this intervention. These issues may have some relevance for FTM transsexuals, especially gay male FTMs.

NOTES

1. Enterprise members report significant changes in their ability to access competent transsexual health care in Boston since 1993. Members actively educate the local medical and social service communities about the needs of FTMs. In addition, the Boston Medical Center sponsors a peer-level support group for FTM transsexuals.

2. Cameron, L. (1996). *Body Alchemy: Transsexual Portraits.* San Francisco: Cleis Press.

3. *You Don't Know Dick: Courageous Hearts of Transsexual Men* (1996). Boston, MA: Northern Light/Candance Schermerhorn Production. This film profiles six FTMs, one of whom is a founding member of Enterprise.

4. McFarland, W., Fischer-Ponce, L., and Katz, M. (1995). Repeat negative HIV testing in San Francisco: Magnitude and characteristics. *American Journal of Epidemiology* October: 719-723. This study found that repeat testers are more likely to be gay or bisexual men, and that these individuals are three times more likely to seroconvert in the future.

5. Prieur, A. (1990). Norwegian gay men: Reasons for continued practice of unsafe sex. *AIDS Education and Prevention* 2(2): 111-113.

6. Odets, W. (1995). *In the Shadow of the Epidemic: Being HIV-Negative in the Age of AIDS.* Durham, NC: Duke University Press, pp. 26-39.

7. Odets, W. (1995). Why we stopped doing primary prevention for gay men in 1985. *AIDS and Public Policy Journal* 10(1): 3-8.

8. Hein, D., Beverley, G., Longo, V., and Burak, M. (1995). A short-term support and education group for HIV-negative gay and bisexual men. Boston: Boston Public Health Commission and Fenway Community Health Center. Unpublished.

9. Brauer, S. (1990). The HIV-infected individual: Group work as a rite of passage. *Smith College Studies in Social Work* 60(3): 233-243.

10. Namaste, V. (1999). HIV/AIDS and female-to-male transsexuals and transvestites: Results from a needs assessment in Québec. *International Journal of Transgenderism* 3 (1-2) (Special Issue on Transgender and HIV: Risks, Prevention, and Care): 1.

11. The flyer was created by an Enterprise member and has the following text: "Dump your fears for an evening of education and soul-searching with Doug Hein,

a professional HIV counselor who runs special workshops dedicated to helping us understand HIV, its impact on our lives, and what we can do."

12. Holzer, J. (1989). Selections from the Living Scenes. Walker Art Center (Sculpture Garden): Minneapolis.

13. Stein, M., Freedberg, K., Sullivan, L., Savetsky, J., Levenson, S., Hingson, R., and Samet, J. (1998). Sexual ethics: Disclosure of HIV-positive status to partners. *Archives of Internal Medicine* 158: 253-257.

14. Rofes, E. (1995). *Reviving the Tribe: Regenerating Gay Men's Sexuality and Culture in the Ongoing Epidemic*. Binghamton, NY: Harrington Park Press, 208.

15. Springer, E. (1991). Effective AIDS prevention with active drug users: The harm reduction model. *Journal of Chemical Dependency Treatment* 4(2): 147-149.

16. Odets, W. (1994). *AIDS education and harm reduction for gay men: Psychological approaches for the 21st century. AIDS & Public Policy Journal* 9(1): 15, quotes from p. 14. Odets promotes AIDS education that "acknowledges the social realities of the epidemic" and is "relatively free of homophobia, misrepresentation, and moralization." He writes, "next among the psychological issues is called 'off line–on line' by Australian psychologist Ron Gold. Put simply, this is the readily observed idea that people exist in different 'states' of consciousness when they are being educated and when they are having sex. In neurophysiological terms, this is the idea that people are educated 'with' their cortexes and have sex—at least substantially—with their brain stems. Gold makes a convincing point: Our education is aimed at the cortex with little regard for how the cortex and brain stem interact *during* sex. Most acculturation and socialization involve 'communication' between these two states of consciousness, and this can be done in the context of AIDS education if we stop educating the cortex as if it were the source of all human feeling and behavior" (emphasis added). Copyright 1994 by University Publishing Group. All rights reserved. Reprinted with permission, <www.upgbooks.com>.

17. Odets, AIDS education and harm reduction for gay men, p. 13.

18. Herdt, G. (1981). *Guardians of the Flutes: Idioms in Masculinity*. New York: McGraw-Hill. Herdt writes about the Sambia tribe in New Guinea in which young boys ingest the semen of older males to acquire male sexual energy and power.

19. Martin, J., and Knox, J. (1995). HIV risk behavior in gay men with unstable self-esteem. *Journal of Gay and Lesbian Social Services* 2(2): 21-41.

20. Devor, H. (1997). *FTM: Female-to-Male Transsexuals in Society*. Bloomington and Indianapolis: Indiana University Press, pp. 467-468. Devor writes about the men in her study, "Within the spheres of their everyday lives, they ceased being transsexuals and became simply men. . . . There were, however, three main areas in which all participants who lived as men were reminded of their transsexualism no matter what their stage of physical transition: in public toilets, in doctors' examination rooms, and in sexual intimacies. These were the areas of their lives wherein they were required to expose those parts of their bodies which proclaimed them to be other than physiologically average males."

21. Prieur, A. (1998). *Mema's House Mexico City: On Transvestites, Queens, and Machos*. Chicago and London: The University of Chicago Press, p. 39. Prieur writes, "Representations form the body, but the body imposes its limits; sexual organs are objective facts that form the representations of gender and the identities. . . .

While bodies are not destinies in any absolute sense, they do form social experiences, and are formed by social experiences." Group members valued experiences with sexual partners who perceived them as male and appreciated their bodies *as they were.* The men reported feeling more self-accepting of their sexual anatomy after such encounters and less focused on anger and grief.

22. Chen, J. (1998). Final report: Evaluation of a three-week support and education program for HIV-negative gay and bisexual men at the Fenway Community Health Center. Boston: Harvard School of Public Health. Unpublished.

Chapter 8

Transgender HIV Prevention: Community Involvement and Empowerment

Walter O. Bockting
B. R. Simon Rosser
Eli Coleman

INTRODUCTION

In collaboration with transgender and HIV/AIDS community organizations, our university-based program developed one of the first HIV prevention education interventions targeting the transgender

The authors thank the following transgender community and HIV/AIDS service organizations for their collaboration: The City of Lakes Crossgender Community, the Minnesota Freedom of Gender Expression, the Aliveness Project, and the Minnesota AIDS Project. Individuals who gave generously of their time and of themselves include Aaron, Celie, Debbie, Dotty/Kevin, Jane, Mira, Sander, and Susan, who served on the planning committee; Kate Bornstein, Steven Grandell, and Paul Stravinsky, who created the video and artwork; the workshop facilitators and panelists; and the focus group, workshop, and evaluation participants. It has been a true privilege working with you. We thank the American Foundation for AIDS Research for funding this project (#100108-12-EG), and Margaret Reinfeld, Susan Leaf, and Charles Fuss for their encouragement and support. Finally, we acknowledge the assistance of Lynn Marasco, Anne Marie Weber-Main, and Libby Frost in preparing the manuscript. Correspondence can be sent to Walter Bockting, PHS, 1300 South Second Street, Suite 180, Minneapolis, MN 55454 (Phone: (612) 625-1500; Fax: (612) 626-8311; E-mail: bockt001@tc.umn.edu.)

population and piloted it in the Minneapolis-St. Paul metropolitan area, Minnesota. Transgender persons are affected by HIV/AIDS, yet virtually no prevention education has been provided (Bockting, Robinson, and Rosser, 1998a). Therefore, we developed a psychoeducational workshop based on the Health Belief Model, the Eroticizing Safer Sex approach to HIV prevention, and principles of personal and community empowerment. Community involvement was key to the success of this project. We offer this experience as a case study of collaboration between a university and community organizations.

"Transgender" is an umbrella term that refers to people who cross or transcend culturally defined categories of gender. They include crossdressers or transvestites (those who desire to wear clothing associated with another sex), male-to-female and female-to-male transsexuals (those who desire or have undergone hormone therapy and/or sex reassignment surgery), transgenderists (those who live in the gender role associated with another sex without desiring sex reassignment surgery), bigender persons (those who identify as both man and woman), drag queens and kings (usually gay men and lesbian women who "do drag" and dress up in, respectively, women's and men's clothes), and female and male impersonators (males who impersonate women and females who impersonate men). Minnesota has a large transgender population due to the availability of transgender-specific health care (Hastings, 1969; Bockting, 1997a; Bockting and Coleman, 1992). Minnesota also was the first state in the United States to specifically include transgender people in human rights legislation (Human Rights Act, 1993).

Historically, the various subgroups of this diverse population have not always cooperated or felt comfortable with one another. For example, male-to-female transsexuals generally distanced themselves from cross-dressers because they believed that, unlike themselves, cross-dressers are "just into the clothes and don't genuinely feel like women." Postoperative transsexuals distanced themselves from preoperative transsexuals in order to blend in with society as "new," no longer transsexual women and men. Heterosexually identified transsexuals and cross-dressers separated themselves from gay-identified drag queens and lesbian-identified drag kings. A hierarchy existed in which those who conformed most to nontransgender members of the desired gender were at the top of the pecking order, and those who conformed least at the bottom. Homophobia, transphobia, and shame reinforced these divisions. As with other marginalized groups, transgender people turned oppression inward and infighting was common, making for a fragmented community.

Subgroups defined on the basis of these divisions congregated in separate quarters and founded corresponding community organizations. The City of Lakes Crossdressers Club (CLCC) was founded in 1984 by cross-dressers who met through association with our outpatient mental health clinic. They started to meet for support and socializing at private homes and later in a hotel. In 1988 several members of the CLCC founded a sister organization, the Minnesota Freedom of Gender Expression, which met at a community center. Female impersonators and drag queens gathered at a local gay and lesbian nightclub and, in 1990, formed a chapter of the International Court System, an organization creating cultural, charitable, and recreational activities for drag queens, impersonators, and their partners and friends and named it the Imperial Sovereign Court of the Ice Castle.

In the 1990s, in the context of a paradigm shift toward affirmation of transgender identity and coming out (Bockting, 1997b; Bolin, 1994; Stone, 1991), the boundaries between these subgroups and divisions within the transgender community began to blur. Transgender people gained greater visibility, organized and empowered themselves, and sought coalitions with the gay, lesbian, and bisexual communities. In 1992, in Minnesota, this was reflected in the new name of the Gay and Lesbian Pride Festival: it became the Gay, Lesbian, Bisexual, and Transgender Pride Festival (see Figure 8.1). The City of Lakes Crossdressers Club became more inclusive of transsexual people, changed its name to the City of Lakes Crossgender Community, and moved its meetings to a local HIV/AIDS service organization. The Minnesota Freedom of Gender Expression began to meet at the offices of the Gay and Lesbian Action Council. Consistent with this paradigm shift and trend in community building, we decided to bring representatives of the various subgroups and community organizations together under the transgender umbrella to initiate targeted HIV prevention.

The rationale for community involvement in our HIV prevention project was based on the belief that "the most effective center of gravity for health promotion is the community" (Kreuter, 1992 p.136). Community involvement ensures acceptability, appropriateness, and relevance of the intervention to the target population, and evidence suggests that people are more committed to initiating and upholding changes that they help design or adapt to their own purposes or circumstances (Wong, Alsagoff, and Koh, 1992). Furthermore, we shared the belief that fostering a sense of ownership raises the credi-

FIGURE 8.1. Logo Illustrating the Inclusion of the Transgender Community in the Twin Cities Pride Festival

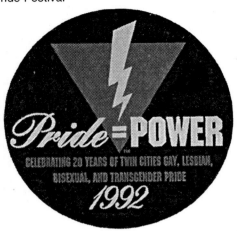

bility of the prevention education message, promotes self-efficacy, and creates community norms that support protective behaviors (Corby, Enguidanos, and Kay, 1996; Mantell and DiVittis, 1990; Person and Cotton, 1996; Simons et al., 1996). To facilitate community involvement, we built on existing relationships between the university and local transgender community and HIV/AIDS service organizations.

Collaboration between community and researchers has been emphasized strongly in the second decade of the AIDS epidemic (e.g., Adrien et al., 1996; Bouie, 1993; House and Walker, 1993; Mantell and DiVittis, 1990; Molbert, Boyer, and Shafer, 1993). The best-known example is the Centers for Disease Control's HIV Community Planning Process, in which U.S. state health departments share the responsibility for identifying and prioritizing HIV prevention needs with representatives of the communities for whom the services are intended (Valdiserri, Aultman, and Curran, 1995). Among the principles that guide this collaboration are these: (1) differences in background, perspective, and experience are essential and valued, (2) roles and responsibilities are clarified at the outset, and policies and procedures for resolving disputes and avoiding conflicts are developed proactively, (3) resources are allocated for community involvement, and (4) shared priority setting is based on an accurate needs assessment, a firm scientific basis for intervention, consumer characteristics and values, and evaluation findings. Challenges in this partnership between community representatives, scientists, prevention workers, and health officials include the complexity of participatory processes, the potential for conflict to decrease administrative efficiency, and the mistrust in marginalized communities of government, scientists, and health authorities. In working with the transgender community—a community even more marginalized than the gay, lesbian, and bisexual communities—we committed ourselves to these challenges and set out to foster involvement and empowerment.

Personal and community empowerment has been shown to positively affect HIV risk reduction. Effective interventions provide HIV prevention education in a context that promotes self-efficacy and affirms self-esteem and pride (DiClemente and Wingood, 1995; Kelly, 1995). The pedagogy of Freire (1970) has guided empowerment approaches in HIV prevention (e.g., Cranston, 1992; Ferreira-Pinto and Ramos, 1995). Educators often define and control the content of the intervention to be delivered to passive participants; Freire argued that participants know their own realities better than anyone else and should be actively engaged in their own education. Fundamental to his approach is the process of raising consciousness among participants through a critical dialogue out of which change and growth emerge. To facilitate empowerment, we involved a core group of community representatives in the development of the intervention, used focus groups, trained peer educators, and included a segment on empowerment in the workshop curriculum.

Establishment of a core group, usually in the form of an advisory board or task force, has been widely applied in HIV prevention. A core group of community leaders, key health professionals, and members of the target population provides input throughout the program development process and shares in making decisions, prioritizing prevention needs, reviewing intervention materials, and disseminating information about the program to potential participants. As the group becomes more invested in the project, core group members who endorse the intervention secure trust and community support (e.g., Bouie, 1993; House and Walker, 1993; Kegeles, Hays, and Coates, 1996; Mantell and DiVittis, 1990). Focus groups, a method that originated in market research, involve members of the target community to qualitatively assess prevention needs, to evaluate the sensitivity and appropriateness of intervention materials, and to obtain suggestions on logistics of program implementation (Mantell and DiVittis, 1990).

Training peer educators to deliver interventions is empowering in more than one way. Peer educators have the opportunity to develop and practice prevention skills. Through their similarities with program participants, they more easily gain participants' attention and respect, promote feelings of self-efficacy through positive role modeling, and intervene on the level of peer norms, creating the expectation that safer sex and safer needle practices are socially accepted and valued. In addition, education by peers who are living with HIV/AIDS has the potential to enhance perceived susceptibility to HIV infection (McKusick, Hortsman, and Coates, 1985; Kelly, 1995). Peer education has been shown to be effective in targeting gay men (Kelly et al., 1991; Kelly et al., 1993), youth (Baldwin, 1995; Kegeles, Hays, and Coates, 1996; Rickert, Jay, and Gottlieb, 1991), women (DiClemente and Wingood, 1995; Kauth et al., 1993; Stevens, 1994), sex workers (O'Reilly and Piot, 1996), and injection drug users (Simons et al., 1996).

We will first describe community involvement in each phase of program development—planning, needs assessment, recruitment, intervention, evaluation, celebration, and replication—then discuss the impact of our project on community building and the lessons we learned, and conclude with recommendations for future collaboration between community organizations and university faculty.

PLANNING

Representatives of the transgender community, the collaborating community organizations, and the university-based investigators formed a planning committee that included preoperative and postoperative male-to-female and female-to-male transsexuals, a transgenderist, a bigender cross-dresser, a transgender sex worker, and a female impersonator/drag queen and a transexual both living with AIDS. Committee members reflected a spectrum of sexual orientation, relationship status, and ethnic identification. Bringing these representatives with varying experiences of identity and sexuality together served to unite them in the fight against AIDS, to enable the community to take ownership of the project, and to tailor intervention and evaluation strategies to the characteristics and needs of the target population. Tasks were divided into three subcommittees, focusing on (1) recruitment, (2) intervention, and (3) evaluation, each reporting in biweekly meetings to the full committee. Group process and consensus guided decision making. Committee members were reimbursed for their time.

NEEDS ASSESSMENT

To inform the intervention, we involved members of the target community in a needs assessment through the use of focus groups (Bockting, Robinson, and Rosser, 1998a). We recruited participants through advertisements in general community newspapers, transgender organizations' newsletters, and personal networks of planning committee members. We conducted four focus groups with a total of nineteen transgender persons (ten transsexuals, six cross-dressers, two transgenderists, and one drag queen/female impersonator), four of them living with HIV/AIDS, according to a method developed by Krueger (1988). Planning committee members helped develop interview questions, focusing on four main areas (1) impact of HIV/AIDS on transgender persons, (2) risk factors, (3) information and services needed, and (4) recruitment strategies. Results were reviewed with the planning committee and incorporated in the intervention.

Focus group findings confirmed the importance of community involvement. Participants suggested the use of transgender role models (e.g., peer educators, transgender-identified health providers, transgender celebrities) to raise the credibility of prevention messages. Participants stressed the value of bringing people together in an environment where it is safe to express their transgender identities; they felt this would be an incentive to attend and serve to combat isolation and alleviate shame stemming from social stigmatization. They recommended that the intervention affirm transgender identity, improve self-esteem, foster a sense of community, and emphasize that life is worth living. Participants suggested that building community based on commonalities among subgroups of the transgender population be balanced with sensitivity to individual differences.

We discovered that the focus groups facilitated community involvement beyond the obvious purpose of gathering useful information directly from members of the target community; they also encouraged the community to become invested in the project. A number of focus group participants became advocates for the project, encouraging others to participate. Half of the focus group participants attended the intervention, and several of them took an active part. For example, participants living with HIV/AIDS volunteered to serve on a panel and share their stories with workshop participants.

RECRUITMENT

The needs assessment focus groups generated several suggestions for recruitment of workshop participants, including advertisements eroticizing safer sex, personal networking, street outreach, and incentives such as food and money. The planning committee reviewed these suggestions and decided to use the following: advertisements and short articles in newsletters, magazines, and community newspapers; posters in locations frequented by the target population; personal and street outreach using wallet-sized cards with pertinent information; announcements on a local transgender computer bulletin board called Carolyn's Closet; and distribution of flyers to clients of key health providers. Homemade snacks were served during the workshop. Unfortunately, budget constraints did not allow us to pay those who attended the workshop for their participation.

Transgender-identified graphic designers produced a logo and prototypes of advertisements eroticizing safer sex with a transgender image. The planning committee reviewed these prototypes and selected a series of four advertisements that potential participants could identify with, that would attract them to the workshop, and that would simultaneously have a preventive effect by eroticizing safer sex. We faced our first hurdle when the university administration deemed three of the four advertisements inappropriate and too explicit and refused to approve them. This criticism pertained to both the visuals and the text. For example, one ad depicted a transgender person dressed in lingerie with the slogan "Let's get down to basics—hot sex is safer sex"; it was intended to attract, among others, those who cross-dress for sexual excitement (fetishistic cross-dressers). We reached a compromise with a less revealing image and a change in the text: "Let's get down to basics—practice safer sex."

Planning committee members wrote short articles that, along with advertisements, appeared in newsletters of the transgender community organizations they represented. Committee members placed posters—enlarged versions of the advertisements—in nightclubs, adult bookstores, public bathrooms, and other establishments. Committee members also conducted personal and street outreach at club meetings, in bars, and in hangouts and stroll areas of transgender sex workers. To ensure access, promote safety, and provide an opportunity for training, much of this outreach was conducted in pairs of an experienced outreach worker and a transgender peer.

We offered the intervention, a four-hour psychoeducational workshop, three times during the course of six months. After satisfactory recruitment for the first workshop (of the projected fifty, thirty-six transgender persons participated), attendance at the second workshop was disappointing (of the thirty-four registrants, sixteen participated), due in part to the extreme winter weather conditions on the day of the workshop. Evaluation findings of the first two workshops showed that personal outreach accounted for the majority (55 percent) of recruits. Therefore, we increased our outreach efforts, and committee members invited their own personal networks through specially designed invitation cards. Because evaluation findings showed that we had primarily attracted preoperative transsexuals (53 percent) and cross-dressers (21 percent), we added advertisements using such terms as "postop transsexuals," "female impersonators," and "drag queens"—instead of the more general term "transgender"—to appeal directly to specific subgroups of the transgender population. To prevent diluting the primary purpose of attracting people to the workshop, these new advertisements did not attempt to eroticize safer sex. As an extra incentive, planning committee members organized a community celebration immediately following the third workshop. These combined efforts doubled recruitment for the third workshop, proving community involvement is invaluable.

INTERVENTION

The development of the workshop was based on (1) findings from the needs assessment focus groups; (2) twenty-five years of experience in providing Sexual Attitude Reassessment seminars and the Transgender Health Seminar (Held et al., 1974; Lief, 1970; Bockting, 1997a; Bockting and Coleman, 1992); (3) the Health Belief Model and the Eroticizing Safer Sex approach to HIV prevention, and principles of empowerment (Janz and Becker, 1984; Rosenstock, Strecher, and Becker, 1994; Palacios-Jimenez and Shernoff, 1986; Fahlberg et al., 1991); and (4) input from the planning committee. Based on our experience with offering the Sexual Attitude Reassessment seminar and the Transgender Health Seminar to transgender clients, we chose a four-hour workshop format, combining three large-group and two small-group meetings. The first large-group presentation aimed to increase the health beliefs of perceived severity and susceptibility to HIV infection and transmission, followed by a small-group discussion to process feelings and identify personal risk. The second large-group meeting promoted risk reduction and eroticized safer sex, and, consistent with the Sexual Attitude Reassessment seminar's methodology, used sexually explicit videos featuring, whenever possible, transgender persons enjoying sex safely. The second small-group meeting built condom and negotiation skills; participants developed individualized preventon plans. The third and final large-group presentation addressed personal and community empowerment by affirming transgender identity, instilling self-confidence and pride, and fostering a sense of community (see Table 8.1; Bockting, Rosser, and Coleman, 2000). The planning committee created and adapted educational materials to appeal directly to the concerns and HIV risks of the transgender participants.

Community involvement in the workshop curriculum and implementation consisted of the following components.

Peer Education

We recruited two large-group and ten small-group leaders from the target community. A well-respected male-to-female transgenderist who enjoyed a leadership role in the community co-facilitated the large-group presentations with the first author. She served as a role model by relating the presented information to her life as a transgender person and as the parent of a son who died of AIDS. Small-group leaders, who reflected the diversity in sexual identity, ethnicity, age, and relationship status of the target to-male group—preoperative and postoperative male-to-female and female-transsexuals, cross-dressers, transgenderists, bigender persons, drag queens, and female impersonators—attended a day-long training (see Table 8.2). The morning program focused on learning the goals and content of the workshop; increasing comfort in talking about sex; developing sensi-

TABLE 8.1. Workshop Curriculum

First Large-Group Presentation (60 minutes)

Goals
1. To assist participants to be comfortable and receptive
2. To explain the purpose of the workshop and the research project
3. To describe the current scope of the HIV/AIDS epidemic
4. To personalize HIV/AIDS
5. To discuss fears, myths, and special vulnerabilities for transgender persons and their partners

Content
a. Welcome and introductions
b. Explanation of purpose
c. Logistics
d. What is HIV?
e. National and local statistics
f. Personalizing HIV/AIDS:
  • Vignette
  • Personal experience
  • Guided visualization
  • Video
g. Myths and concerns about HIV/AIDS
h. Special vulnerabilities
i. Panel of transgender persons living with HIV/AIDS

First Small-Group Meeting (60 minutes)

Goals
1. To provide a supportive and nonjudgmental place to process fears, concerns, and experiences about HIV/AIDS
2. To identify personal HIV risks
3. To enable open discussion of sexual behavior, substance use, and gender concerns

Content
a. Confidentiality
b. Introductions
c. Emotional reactions and processing
d. Dyad exercise sharing experiences of HIV risk
e. Reasons for unsafe sex: Identify personal HIV risks

Second Large-Group Presentation (45 minutes)

Goals
1. To help participants understand how HIV is transmitted
2. To affirm and eroticize safer sex using an erotopositive and transgender-sensitive framework
3. To educate participants on risk reduction in the use of injection paraphernalia
4. To teach assertiveness skills to insist on safer sex and safer needle practices

Content
a. Introduction to preventing HIV transmission
b. Myths and facts about HIV transmission
c. Making sex fun and safe: Eroticizing safer sex
  • Continuum of sexual risk
  • Safer-sex hints
d. Condom use
e. Sexually explicit videos affirming safer sex
f. Video: Safer needle practices
g. Sexual assertiveness and negotiation
  • Reasons for unsafe sex
  • Need for assertiveness
  • Personal risk and prevention plan

TABLE 8.1 *(continued)*

Second Small-Group Meeting (50 minutes)

Goals	Content
1. To practice condom use skills	a. Dyad condom exercise
2. To rehearse negotiation skills through role-play	b. Fish bowl role-play negotiating safer sex
3. To develop an individualized prevention plan	c. Dyad role-plays negotiating safer sex or safer needle use
	d. Individualize prevention plan with help from the group
	e. Eroticize own sexual behavior
	f. Concrete commitment to practice safer behaviors

Third Large-Group Presentation (20 minutes)

Goals	Content
1. To provide referral for HIV testing	a. HIV testing: Transgender-sensitive testing sites
2. To respond to (medical) questions	b. Questions and answers by a transsexual physician
3. To foster personal and community empowerment	c. Pride = Power: Personal and community empowerment
	d. Ritual facilitated by a transsexual community activist
	e. Video: *Condoms Are a Girl's Best Friend*

TABLE 8.2. Small-Group Leaders' Training Curriculum

9:00 a.m.	Welcome and introductions	
9:30 a.m.	Explanation of goals and content of the intervention	Overview of workshop curriculum
10:00 a.m.	Talking about sex	Group exercise: Sexual words Dyad exercise: Sexual language
10:20 a.m.	Break	
10:30 a.m.	Transgender identity and sexuality: Information, attitudes, and values	Lecture, video, and discussion

11:15 a.m.	HIV/AIDS: Information, attitudes, and values	Lecture, video, and discussion
11:50 a.m.	Safer sex and risk reduction in the use of injection paraphernalia	Lecture, video, and discussion
12:30 p.m.	Lunch	
1:30 p.m.	Group facilitation skills: 1. Ground rules: Confidentiality, respect, boundaries 2. Facilitation skills: Modeling, interaction, guidance 3. Specific techniques: Talking about sex, active listening, probing, summarizing	Lecture and handout
2:00 p.m.	First small-group simulation	Facilitator role rotates
3:00 p.m.	Break	
3:15 p.m.	Facilitating exercises and role-plays	Lecture and handout
3:45 p.m.	Second small-group simulation	Facilitator role rotates
4:35 p.m.	Wrap up	Questions and discussion
5:00 p.m.	Adjourn	

tivity to the diversity in transgender identity and sexuality; increasing HIV/AIDS knowledge and desirable attitudes; and understanding risk behavior, safer sex, and risk reduction in the use of injection paraphernalia. The afternoon program focused on developing facilitation skills in group discussion, exercises, and role-play. Through small-group simulations, peer educators rehearsed their skills.

Video Clip Personalizing HIV/AIDS

To involve a transgender celebrity as a role model, we invited transsexual performing artist Kate Bornstein to conceive a video clip to personalize HIV/AIDS. Kate met with a group of community members to learn about their perceptions of how HIV/AIDS applies to them as transgender people. In writing the script, she incorporated themes and comments that surfaced during this meeting. A local transgender video artist filmed and edited a nine-minute infomercial that featured, along with Kate, three local people (a male-to-female transsexual, a female-to-male transsexual, and a drag queen/female impersonator), each playing a transgender person uniquely at risk for HIV. Among the HIV cofactors addressed in this video are identity confusion or conflict, shame and isolation, secrecy, and fear of discovery and rejection. Toward the end of the video, Kate affirms participants' self-worth and empowers them to confront their HIV risk (Bockting, Grandell, and Bornstein, 1992):

> Trust yourself. Trust yourself to know that you're a good and decent human being. Trust yourself to know that your life counts in this world. Trust yourself to protect yourself around HIV and AIDS. And the next time a voice comes up and tells you to be silent, please remember how very loved you are in the scheme of this world; and speak up in spite of the voice that might silence you. You're my family. I can't tell you how glad I am that you're at this workshop. Please be proud of yourself. Please speak up about AIDS and HIV. Please keep on living.

Panel of Transgender Persons Living with HIV/AIDS

We accepted the offer of focus group participants with HIV/AIDS to make a panel presentation during the workshop. Two individuals, a transsexual and a drag queen/female impersonator, introduced themselves and engaged in a question-and-answer session with workshop participants. We asked panel members to focus on the personal, on their adjustment, identities, and sexuality, and to avoid intellectualizing and recounting lengthy hospital stories. For example:

> Q: Which, if any, of your cross-gender issues affected your contracting the HIV virus?

> A: I think, for me, it would be being in denial of my transsexualism for a long time, having to repress that and having to repress my sexuality, feeling really ashamed about the whole thing. It is really easy to have unsafe sex when you feel that way, because those feelings of shame can override anything, because they are very strong. The biggest thing that anyone can do is deal with that, accepting themselves and loving themselves, knowing that they're worth it, you know, all of that.

Q: Does your family know?

A: My family knows. My mother never accepted that I have AIDS. She can't understand that her eldest son is really a female. My brother says it's a bunch of bullshit. My sister is real supportive. My sister says she doesn't know why it took me so long to decide to grow up to be a woman. My sister is my biggest support.

The panel presentation was so successful that several other workshop participants also living with HIV/AIDS volunteered to be on the panel during subsequent interventions.

Sexually Explicit Videos Featuring Transgender Models

During the second large-group presentation designed to promote risk reduction, we showed sexually explicit videos eroticizing safer sex. Previous research demonstrated that such videos reinforce behavior change (Quadland et al., 1987). Although finding educational videos portraying transgender persons having sex was difficult, we managed to locate a video of a female-to-male transsexual and a nontransgender female partner practicing safer sex (Jaccoma, Armstrong, and Sprinkle, 1990).

Transgender Physician

We invited a female-to-male transsexual physician to discuss HIV testing and answer medical questions. We were amazed by the number of medical questions, suggesting that future interventions should address medical aspects more extensively. Questions specific to transgender concerns included "What are the effects of hormone therapy on HIV risk and disease progression?" and "What is the risk of HIV infection through electrolysis?"

Transgender Community Activist

In the third large-group presentation, a male-to-female transsexual local politician and community activist fostered community and empowerment. She stressed the commonalities among subgroups of the transgender community, creating a sense of unity. She affirmed the coalition of the gay, lesbian, and bisexual communities and the transgender community by reminding participants of the role drag queens played in the 1969 Stonewall Rebellion (which marked the beginning of America's gay rights movement), and by pointing out their shared struggle for social acceptance, for human rights, and against AIDS. She facilitated a ritual. As participants stood in a circle, she wrapped a red ribbon around their hands, nurturing feelings of solidarity, affirming transgender identity and sexuality, and instilling self-confidence and gender pride. All participants kept a piece of the ribbon to remind them of being part of a community and a future worth living for.

Video Affirming Transgender Expression and Promoting Condom Use

To end the workshop, we showed a video titled *Condoms Are a Girl's Best Friend,* a parody of Marilyn Monroe's song "Diamonds Are a Girl's Best Friend," performed by a female impersonator, and interspersed with scenes of transgender persons and their partners (Lane and Kay, 1991).

EVALUATION

We assessed community support, participant satisfaction, and changes in participants' AIDS knowledge, attitudes, and HIV risk behaviors both quantitatively and qualitatively (Bockting, Robinson, and Rosser, 1998b; Bockting, Rosser, and Scheltema, 1999). Quantitative evaluation consisted of comparisons between participants' responses on preworkshop, postworkshop, and two-month follow-up questionnaires. The evaluation subcommittee of the planning committee drafted the questionnaires, which were pilot tested and reviewed by the entire committee for cultural sensitivity and relevance. It was particularly rewarding to free questions from conventional assumptions of sex and gender in order to account for the unique anatomies and realities of transgender persons. The outcome was an instrument with clear, descriptive questions that reflected the notion that the risk of HIV is behavior based and not dependent on gender or sexual orientation. For further clarity, the committee defined a list of transgender-specific and other key terms to guide respondents.

During this process, tension between community representatives and evaluators on the planning committee arose. Several community representatives felt strongly that the service we were providing—the HIV prevention intervention—should not be overshadowed by the research component, the questionnaire evaluation. They argued that too obtrusive an evaluation process would make participants feel like guinea pigs and compromise the intervention by affecting participants' trust and comfort. Others pointed out the value of evaluation of our model program for future interventions and for the long-term welfare of the community. Resolution of this conflict benefited from the community and research expertise represented on the committee, resulting in a substantially shorter questionnaire.

Planning committee members assisted in data collection by staffing the evaluation booth at the workshop, together with investigators, providing an opportunity for training in administering program evaluation. After analyzing the data, investigators discussed with the planning committee aggregate results and their implications for future intervention and research. Results showed an increase in AIDS knowledge and in positive attitudes toward AIDS, sex, safer sex, and condoms. Results also showed that participants socialized more than before with transgender persons in the months following the workshop, suggesting a decrease in isolation and a positive impact on community building. Participant satisfaction with the workshop was high (Bockting, Rosser, and Scheltema, 1999; Bockting, Rosser, and Coleman, 2000).

Qualitative evaluation consisted of a focus group of randomly selected workshop participants. Questions focused on intervention impact, satisfaction, and suggestions for improvement. Results indicated a dramatic increase in AIDS awareness, with participants teaching their respective communities what they learned in the workshop. They reported many conversations about safer sex with friends and family, and on the Internet. The panel presentation of transgender persons living with HIV/AIDS turned out to be powerful in raising perceived severity and susceptibility. The involvement of peer educators as small-group leaders was well received; participants valued the leaders' skills in making people feel comfortable and safe to open up. Participants showed great enthusiasm for more targeted HIV prevention education to protect and care for their community. They recommended that future prevention education take a more contextual approach, integrating HIV prevention in efforts to improve overall health and psychosocial adjustment. Participants asked for a further tailoring of intervention strategies to the different subgroups of the transgender population and wanted to hold the workshop at community sites. The focus group itself seemed to have a preventive effect;

during the discussion, participants reinforced prevention messages for one another (Bockting, Robinson, and Rosser, 1998b).

We involved planning committee members in disseminating evaluation findings to the community. We distributed a program manual outlining the intervention and evaluation findings to interested community members (Bockting, Rosser, and Coleman, 1993). Together with the first author, transgender community representatives shared findings with family physicians at the university, and with researchers, funders, prevention workers, and representatives from communities nationwide at the HIV Prevention Research Development Meeting in conjunction with the Seventeenth National Lesbian and Gay Health Conference and the Thirteenth Annual AIDS/HIV Forum.

CELEBRATION

Although the impetus for the community celebration following the third workshop was to boost recruitment, it also served to acknowledge the successful completion of our project. Planning committee members organized the gathering at their regular meeting site, which had shifted during the course of the project to a gay, lesbian, bisexual, and now transgender nightclub. All workshop participants, staff, and the wider transgender community were invited. During this celebration, we honored planning committee members and peer educators for their contributions and presented them with an AIDS ribbon pin. The female impersonator with HIV/AIDS who served on the committee provided entertainment. This was a proud and well-attended community-building event.

REPLICATION

Upon completion of our one-year project, we discussed future endeavors with the planning committee. We agreed to shift further the responsibility for the intervention to the community, with university staff retreating into an advisory role. One committee member offered the workshop at the annual convention of the International Foundation for Gender Education in 1996. Attended by representatives of national and international transgender communities, this workshop had a twofold purpose: to address HIV for convention attendees and to give them an experience to build on in implementing HIV prevention efforts in their own communities. We trained two new large-group leaders, a cross-dresser and a female-to-male transsexual, and fifteen transgender-identified small-group leaders to facilitate the workshop. Additional video material was incorporated (The Gender Centre, 1995). This particular workshop was dedicated to two transgender community activists, Louis Sullivan and Jennifer Richards, both of whom died of AIDS. As an outgrowth of this event, the first author was invited to write an article for *Transgender Tapestry,* the magazine of the International Foundation for Gender Education, which enjoys a large worldwide distribution (Bockting, 1996).

Since the completion of our project, we have received numerous requests for the program manual. This led to the establishment of an international network of grassroots initiatives in transgender HIV prevention through which we have shared intervention materials; collaborative projects are under way.

DISCUSSION

Impact on Community Building

Our project had a positive impact on community building. We brought representatives of the various segments of the heretofore fragmented transgender community together and united them in the fight against AIDS. The planning committee and peer educators became a team. Transgender participants living with HIV/AIDS started an informal support group. Workshop participants from various backgrounds and with various transgender identities and sexualities bonded during the intervention and celebration.

Throughout and following our project, relationships between the various subgroups of the transgender community have strengthened. The City of Lakes Crossgender Community moved with the Minnesota Freedom of Gender Expression to a local gay, lesbian, bisexual, and now also transgender nightclub. The Imperial Sovereign Court of the Ice Castle crowned a transsexual woman as their empress, and the planning committee member who identified as a transgenderist (the former president of the City of Lakes Crossgender Community) joined the court and performed as a female impersonator. Three new transgender community organizations formed. One planning committee member founded the Gender Education Center, the first local transgender community organization to receive funds for sensitizing, among others, health providers and prevention workers to transgender issues. Transsexuals founded the New Men and Women of Minnesota; Tri-Ess, a national organization of cross-dressers and their partners, formed a local chapter. In addition, drag kings and male impersonators gathered at Vulva Riot, a local cabaret. These groups now maintain unprecedented cooperative relationships and together hosted the convention of the International Foundation for Gender Education—Minnesota Pride 1996—where their coalition with the gay, lesbian, and bisexual community was cemented in a keynote address by Melinda Paras, executive director of the National Gay and Lesbian Task Force. Important differences between these groups notwithstanding, they all cross or transcend culturally defined categories of gender. Together, they are stronger in the pursuit of equality and human rights.

Lessons Learned

Although community involvement in our project built on longstanding relationships with the local transgender community, the target group's distrust of health researchers, practitioners, and policymakers indeed surfaced. Similar to communities of color and the gay, lesbian, and bisexual community, transgender people have not always felt that authorities are on their side. As one transgender person said during our needs assessment, "My contention is that the AIDS crisis was allowed to happen by the U.S. government, the result being that sexual minorities are especially vulnerable to contracting this disease and dying. Hence, AIDS is society's punishment for being queer." The transgender community has had its share of negative experiences with researchers and health providers. For example, research was used in 1979 to discontinue sex reassignment services at Johns Hopkins University (Meyer and Reter, 1979; Money, 1991). Transgender persons report many negative experiences with health care providers based on ignorance and prejudice. Moreover, the medicalization of transvestism and transsexualism and the gatekeeping role of mental health professionals without whose written recommendation a physician cannot initiate hormone therapy or perform sex reassignment surgery are subjects of growing tension between providers and consumers (Levine et al., 1998; Bolin, 1988, 1994).

Since we are the main providers of sex reassignment services in the community, this issue of distrust was especially challenging for us. Although we consciously avoided dual relationships, a member of our planning committee and small-group leader, while continuing to participate in the HIV prevention project, rallied a community protest publicly denouncing our clinical services. Another committee member temporarily resigned out of solidarity with the protesters. Because of our obligation to protect client confidentiality and our desire not to aggravate the situation, we initially responded cautiously. As the conflict continued to escalate, we intervened with the planning committee, with individual members of the community, and eventually in a public forum. The crisis was not resolved until we articulated clearly what we stood for, set limits with regard to the accusations leveled against us, and negotiated boundaries in relationships with community members. We discovered that the community perceived our initial reserved response as uncaring. We regretted that we had not defined our working relationship and boundaries more clearly at the outset and agreed on how to handle conflict, as recommended by others (Adrien et al., 1996; Valdiserri, Aultman, and Curran, 1995). Working through this conflict forced both parties to examine issues from each other's perspective, recognizing the potential and limits of collaboration, ultimately leading to a deepening of mutual respect and trust.

RECOMMENDATIONS FOR FUTURE COLLABORATION

Make a Commitment to Reciprocal Collaboration

Successful, empowering community-university collaboration must be truly reciprocal. This requires a commitment on both sides to communicate, listen, respect each other's goals and values, and share in decision making. We recommend involving a core group of community representatives earlier than we did, in the proposal stage of the project, or, ideally, as an early, ongoing forum to identify and address community health needs. Group process allows Freire's critical dialogue to occur; group consensus allows participants to share in decision making. At the outset, define and agree upon roles and responsibilities, along with ways to deal with conflict (e.g., keeping and resolving conflict within the group so as not to jeopardize the project).

Strive for Community-Based Intervention

We recommend that the intervention be designed and implemented as much as possible by the community. University-based interventionists can help mobilize the community, secure funding, apply relevant scientific knowledge, and facilitate skill development (e.g., by training peer educators). If the community lacks the infrastructure to initiate targeted prevention education, the university should not hesitate to take the lead. Once the community has gained sufficient cohesiveness, the university could fall back to a consulting or advisory position, shifting responsibility to the community.

Educate and Involve the Community in Research and Evaluation

Community-based interventions can benefit greatly from adequate formative and evaluation research. Epidemiological research is often needed to justify funding for prevention education; interventions informed by group-specific needs assessments are more likely to be successful; and evaluation can document effectiveness and provide helpful information for program improvement. We recommend that university-based researchers educate community representatives about these benefits and actively involve them in research and evaluation, while taking care to balance research and intervention priorities so that evaluation does not overshadow intervention.

CONCLUSION

We believe that, as a result of our collaboration, both the university and the transgender community have grown (Bockting, 1993). We learned that affirmation of transgender identity, peer support, and empowerment are key in promoting transgender health; we now stress these elements also in our clinical services. The transgender community has come together and solidified its coalition with the gay, lesbian, and bisexual community. Aware of their HIV risk and supported by university faculty, transgender community members petitioned successfully for a seat on the State Commissioner's Task Force on HIV Prevention, the guiding body of Minnesota's HIV prevention community planning process. The seat that they proudly claimed as their own was named in honor of a transsexual member of our planning committee, Celie Mahu Edwards, who died of AIDS. We look forward to continuing collaboration to promote community health.

REFERENCES

Adrien, A., Godin, G., Cappon, P., Singer, S.M., Maticka-Tyndale, E., and Willms, D. (1996). Overview of the Canadian study on the determinants of ethnoculturally specific behaviours related to HIV/AIDS. *Canadian Journal of Public Health,* 87(Supplement 1), S4-S10.

Baldwin, J. (1995). Using peer education approaches in HIV/AIDS programs for youth: A review of the literature. *The Peer Facilitator Quarterly,* 12(3), 34-37.

Bockting, W.O. (1993). [Letter to the editor]. *Chrysalis Quarterly,* 1(6), 5-7.

Bockting, W.O. (1996). The seven important things transgender people should know about AIDS. *Transgender Tapestry,* 76, 30-38.

Bockting, W.O. (1997a). The assessment and treatment of gender dysphoria. *Directions in Clinical and Counseling Psychology,* 7(11), 1-23.

Bockting, W.O. (1997b). Transgender coming out: Implications for the clinical management of gender dysphoria. In B. Bullough, V.L. Bullough, and J. Elias (Eds.), *Gender blending* (pp. 48-52). Amherst, NY: Prometheus Books.

Bockting, W.O. and Coleman, E. (1992). A comprehensive approach to the treatment of gender dysphoria. In W.O. Bockting and E. Coleman (Eds.), *Gender dysphoria: Interdisciplinary approaches in clinical management* (pp. 131-155). Binghamton, NY: The Haworth Press.

Bockting, W.O. (Producer), Grandell, S. (Editor), and Bornstein, K. (Script writer) (1992). *Gender defender with AIDS-be-gone infomercial* [Video]. Minneapolis, MN: Program in Human Sexuality.

Bockting, W.O., Robinson, B.E., and Rosser, B.R.S. (1998a). Transgender HIV prevention: A qualitative needs assessment. *AIDS Care,* 10(4), 505-526.

Bockting, W.O., Robinson, B.E., and Rosser, B.R.S. (1998b). Transgender HIV prevention: Qualitative evaluation of a model prevention education program. *Journal of Sex Education and Therapy,* 23(2), 125-133.

Bockting, W.O., Rosser, B.R.S., and Coleman, E. (1993). *Transgender HIV prevention program manual.* Minneapolis, MN: Program in Human Sexuality.

Bockting, W.O., Rosser, B.R.S., and Coleman, E. (2000). Transgender HIV prevention: A model education workshop. *Journal of the Gay and Lesbian Medical Association,* 4(4), 175-183.

Bockting, W.O., Rosser, B.R.S., and Scheltema, K. (1999). Transgender HIV prevention: Implementation and evaluation of a workshop. *Health Education Research; Theory and Practice,* 14(2), 177-183.

Bolin, A. (1988). *In search of Eve: Transsexual rites of passage.* South Hadley, MA: Bergin and Garvey Publishers.

Bolin, A. (1994). Transcending and transgendering: Male-to-female transsexuals, dichotomy and diversity. In G. Herdt (Ed.). *Third sex, third gender: Beyond sexual dimorphism in culture and history.* (pp. 477-485) New York: Zone Books.

Bouie, J., Jr. (1993). A community-organization model for the prevention of alcohol and other drug abuse, HIV transmission, and AIDS among African Americans. In National Conference on Preventing and Treating Alcohol and Other Drug Abuse, HIV Infection, and AIDS in Black Communities, *The second national conference on preventing and treating alcohol and other drug abuse, HIV infection, and AIDS in black communities: From advocacy to action* (pp. 189-204). Rockville, MD: U.S. Department of Health and Human Services, Public Health Service, Substance Abuse and Mental Health Services Administration, Center for Substance Abuse Prevention (CSAP prevention monograph 13).

Corby, N.H., Enguidanos, S.M., and Kay, L.S. (1996). Development and use of role model stories in a community level HIV risk reduction intervention. *Public Health Reports,* 3 (Supplement 1), S4-S8.

Cranston, K. (1992). HIV education for gay, lesbian, and bisexual youth: Personal risk, personal power, and the community of conscience. *Journal of Homosexuality,* 22(3/4), 247-259.

DiClemente, R.J. and Wingood, G.M. (1995). A randomized controlled trial of an HIV sexual risk-reduction intervention for young African-American women. *JAMA,* 274(16), 1271-1276.

Fahlberg, L.L., Poulin, A.L., Girdano, D.A., and Dusek, D.E. (1991). Empowerment as an emerging approach in health education. *Journal of Health Education,* 22(3), 185-193.

Ferreira-Pinto, J.B. and Ramos, R. (1995). HIV/AIDS prevention among female sexual partners of injection drug users in Ciudad Juarez, Mexico. *AIDS Care,* 7(4), 477-488.

Freire, P. (1970). *Pedagogy of the oppressed.* New York: Continuum.

Gender Centre, The (Producer). (1995). *Shattered illusions* [Video]. Petersham, Australia: The Gender Centre.

Hastings, D.W. (1969). Inauguration of a research project on transsexualism in a university medical center. In R. Green and J. Money (Eds.), *Transsexualism and sex reassignment* (pp. 243-251). Baltimore, MD: Johns Hopkins Press.

Held, J., Cournoyer, C., Held, C., and Chilgren, R. (1974). Sexual attitude reassessment: A training seminar for health professionals. *Minnesota Medicine,* 57, 925-928.

House, R.M. and Walker, C.M. (1993). Preventing AIDS via education. *Journal of Counseling and Development,* 71 (January/February), 282-289.

Human Rights Act, Chapter 363, Department of Human Rights, Minnesota Statutes (1993).

Jaccoma, A., Armstrong, J., and Sprinkle, A. (1990). *Linda, Les, and Annie: The first female-to-male transsexual love story* [Video].

Janz, K. and Becker, M.H. (1984). The Health Belief Model: A decade later. *Health Education Quarterly,* 11(1), 1-47.

Kauth, M.R., Christoff, K.A., Sartor, J., and Sharp, S. (1993). HIV sexual risk reduction among college women: Applying a peer influence model. *Journal of College Student Development,* 34 (September), 346-351.

Kegeles, S.M., Hays, R.B., and Coates, T.J. (1996). The Mpowerment Project: A community-level HIV prevention intervention for young gay men. *American Journal of Public Health,* 8(86), 1129-1136.

Kelly, J.A. (1995). Advances in HIV/AIDS education and prevention. *Family Relations,* 44, (October) 345-352.

Kelly, J.A., Murphy, D.A., Sikkema, K.J., and Kalichman, S.C. (1993). Psychological interventions to prevent HIV infection are urgently needed: New priorities for behavioral research in the second decade of AIDS. *American Psychologist,* 48(10), 1023-1034.

Kelly, J.A., St. Lawrence, J.S., Diaz, Y.E., Stevenson, L.Y., Hauth, A.C., Brasfield, T.L., Kalichman, S.C., Smith, J.E., and Andrew, M.E. (1991). HIV risk behavior reduction following intervention with key opinion leaders of population: An experimental analysis. *American Journal of Public Health,* 81(2), 168-171.

Kreuter, M.W. (1992). PATCH, its origin, basic concepts, and links to contemporary public health policy. *Journal of Health Education,* 2(3), 135-139.

Krueger, R.A. (1988). *Focus groups: A practical guide for applied research.* Newbury Park, CA: Sage Publications.

Lane, M. (Executive Producer) and Kay, E. C. (Producer and Director) (1991). *Condoms are a girl's best friend* [Video]. Chicago, IL: Memory Lane.

Levine, S.B., Brown, G.R., Coleman, E., Cohen-Kettenis, P.T., Hage, J.J., Van Maasdam, J., Petersen, M., Pfaefflin, F., and Schaefer, L.C. (1998). The standards of care for gender identity disorders. *International Journal of Transgenderism* [Online serial], 2(2). Available <http://www.symposion. com/ijt/ijtc0405.htm>.

Lief, H.I. (1970). Developments in the sex education of the physician. *Journal of the American Medical Association,* 212, 1864-1867.

Mantell, J.E. and DiVittis, A.T. (1990). AIDS prevention programs: The need for evaluation in the context of community partnership. *New Directions for Program Evaluation,* 46 (Summer), 87-98.

McKusick, L., Hortsman, W., and Coates, T.J. (1985). AIDS and the sexual behavior reported by gay men in San Francisco. *American Journal of Public Health,* 7(5), 493-496.

Meyer, J.K. and Reter, D.J. (1979). Sex reassignment follow-up. *Archives of General Psychiatry,* 36 (August), 1010-1015.

Molbert, W., Boyer, C.B., and Shafer, M.B. (1993). Implementing a school-based STD/HIV prevention intervention: Collaboration between a university medical center and an urban school district. *Journal of School Health,* 63(6), 258-261.

Money, J. (1991). Serendipities on the sexological pathway to research in gender identity and sex reassignment. *Journal of Psychology and Human Sexuality,* 4(1), 101-113.

O'Reilly, K.R. and Piot, P. (1996). International perspectives on individual and community approaches to the prevention of sexually transmitted disease and human immunodeficiency virus infection. *The Journal of Infectious Diseases,* 174(Supplement 2), S214-S222.

Palacios-Jimenez, L. and Shernoff, M. (1986). *Facilitators guide to eroticizing safer sex: A psychoeducational workshop approach to safer sex education.* New York: Gay Men's Health Crisis.

Person, B. and Cotton, D. (1996). A model of community mobilization for the prevention of HIV in women and infants. *Public Health Reports,* 3(Supplement 1), 89-98.

Quadland, M., Shattls, W., Schuman, R., Jacobs, R., and D'Eramo, J. (1987). *The 800 men project: A report on the design, implementation, and evaluation of an AIDS prevention and education program.* New York: Gay Men's Health Crisis.

Rickert, V.I., Jay, M.S., and Gottlieb, A. (1991). Effects of a peer-counseled AIDS education program on knowledge, attitudes, and satisfaction of adolescents. *Journal of Adolescent Health,* 12(1), 38-43.

Rosenstock, I.M., Strecher, V.J., and Becker, M.H. (1994). The Health Belief Model and HIV risk behavior change. In R.J. DiClemente and J.L. Peterson (Eds.), *Preventing AIDS: Theories and methods of behavioral interventions* (pp. 5-24). New York: Plenum Press.

Simons, P.Z., Rietmeijer, C.A., Kane, M.S., Guenther-Grey, C., Higgins, D.L., and Cohn, D.L. (1996). Building a peer network for a community level HIV prevention program among injecting drug users in Denver. *Public Health Reports,* 3(Supplement 1), 50-53.

Stevens, P.E. (1994). HIV prevention education for lesbians and bisexual women: A cultural analysis of a community intervention. *Social Science and Medicine,* 39(11), 1565-1578.

Stone, S. (1991). The empire strikes back: A posttranssexual manifesto. In J. Epstein and K. Straub (Eds.), *Body guards: The cultural politics of gender ambiguity.* (pp. 280-304) New York: Routledge.

Valdiserri, R.O., Aultman, T.V., and Curran, J.W. (1995). Community planning: A national strategy to improve HIV prevention programs. *Journal of Community Health,* 20(2), 87-100.

Wong, M.L., Alsagoff, F., and Koh, D. (1992). Health promotion: A further field to conquer. *Singapore Medical Journal,* 33, 341-346.

Chapter 9

Sex, Truth, and Videotape: HIV Prevention at the Gender Identity Project in New York City

Barbara E. Warren

INTRODUCTION

In the videotape produced by the Gender Identity Project of New York City's Lesbian and Gay Community Services Center, *Safe T Lessons: HIV Prevention for the Transgender Communities,* transgender activist Riki Ann Wilchins talks frankly about her own experiences of looking for sex as a rite of passage into womanhood and the risk she would take to be accepted as a desirable female. "You want to be accepted and sex feels like acceptance . . . even for a night, even for fifteen minutes . . . lots of trans people will have unsafe sex to feel desirable, to feel loved, to be validated as a woman or man." Tony Baretto-Neto tells other transsexual men that transitioning to male from a lesbian identity, he never thought of himself as at risk, even though he was trained as a police officer to educate other cops about HIV. Cross-dresser Terri McCorkel tells a story about Joe, who when dressed up as a woman, dares to have erotic experiences, including unprotected sex with a man, that he would not risk doing as Joe.

Imperial Court Empress Philomena, self-identified drag queen, reveals that drag is all about the illusion of being female, and for some drag queens and their partners, using condoms might call too much attention to male genitalia. Peer educator Nora Molina worries about the HIV-positive transsexual sex workers who do not use condoms with their customers in order to make more money, thereby placing themselves at greater risk for secondary infection and other diseases.

All of these issues and more are being discussed and addressed within the HIV prevention and intervention efforts of the Gender Identity Project. Since 1990, the Lesbian and Gay Community Services Center of New York City has been serving transgender persons through the Gender Identity Project (GIP), the first (and still one of the few) transgender peer counseling and empowerment programs in the country. The GIP's constituency includes a wide range of transgender identities: cross-dressers, femme and butch queens, bigenders, drag kings and queens, and transsexuals.

Transgender people, similar to gay men and lesbians, experience prejudice and exclusion from the larger society. In this respect, the Gender Identity Project fits in with the Center's overall mission to protect and preserve lesbian and gay rights and culture. The GIP mirrors the Center's mission in its efforts to provide transgender persons an opportunity to affirm who they are in an atmosphere of self-acceptance, as well as an opportunity to build community. The GIP has developed as primarily a peer-driven peer support project that relies on transgender people to help other transgender people to assess community needs and create support mechanisms. Peer counselors, some of whom are human services professionals, work with other Center staff to deliver individual, group, and other support services. For many recipients, the peer counseling is the first time they encounter a peer who not only shares their experiences but is also a role model for the successful resolution of their gender identity issues.

Although more data on HIV/AIDS in transgender populations are needed, recent studies indicate that the transgender community is at high risk for both substance abuse and HIV (Yates, 1998; Mason, Connors, and Kammerer, 1995). Clements, Kitano, and Marx (1998) found that HIV risk behaviors are common in transgender men and women; that HIV prevalence is higher for the transgender population than for both men who have sex with men and injection drug users in San Francisco; that HIV-infected transgender women continue to engage in high-risk sexual behaviors; and that there is a distinct lack of transgender affirmative services available, even in San Francisco, a city known for its innovative programs. Elifson and colleagues (1993) found a high rate of non-HIV sexually transmitted disease among transgender-identified sex workers, which is correlated with additional risk for HIV transmission. Anecdotal data on the use of shared needles for injection hormones and the need for hormone needle exchange (Positive Health Project, 1998) also indicate that transgender persons are at significant risk for HIV.

PROGRAM PARTICIPANTS

Since its inception, GIP has collected demographic data on program participants. A recent analysis of this data set has helped to inform GIP prevention efforts. The data are unique in that they document a wide variety of variables from 1990 through the present, for a relatively large, nonclinical sample of clients (N = 357) in a community-based setting (Valentine, 1998). Of GIP clients, 55 percent are white, 20 percent are Latino/Latina, 14 percent are African American, and 10 percent report being biracial or multiracial. The mean age for white clients is thirty-six years; for African Americans, thirty-two; and for Latinos/Latinas, twenty-eight. This does not include data on thirteen-to twenty-one-year-olds, who are tracked from the Center's Youth Enrichment Services (YES) program, which reports about 3 percent of young persons in the YES program identifying as transgender.

Data collected on the genders of sexual partners indicate that transgender people are sexually active across the spectrum of sexual orientation, with 45 percent reporting sexual attraction to men, 29 percent reporting sexual attraction to women, and 20 percent reporting bisexual attraction. Substance abuse, a known risk factor for HIV transmission, is high among transgender people, with 27 percent self-reporting alcohol abuse and 24 percent reporting drug abuse, across all ethnic groups and gender identities. This is twice the rate found in the general population and comparable to the higher rate of substance abuse found in the research on the lesbian and gay communities (McKirnan and Peterson, 1989).

HIV status in the earlier years of data collection was poor because nearly half of the sample declined to report their status, and as it was not a requirement of program participation, peer counselors did not pursue the information. With the development of the GIP's HIV prevention education program, HIV training for peer counselors, and greater awareness in the transgender communities about the need for HIV education, more consistent data have been collected recently, with 40 percent reporting HIV-negative status and 6 percent reporting HIV-positive status. The majority of transgender persons do not know their HIV status. As previously described, anecdotal and ethnographic evidence suggest a higher rate of HIV infection in these communities, particularly among sex worker populations. All of these results indicate the need for more intensive HIV-related services directed toward, and available to, transgender populations.

PEER-DRIVEN ASSESSMENT OF NEEDS

The Gender Identity Project's roots in peer education and community building make it an ideal vehicle for HIV education. It is well documented that peer-delivered outreach and education are essential tools to successful HIV prevention and intervention. As previously stated, at the time that the GIP undertook development and implementation of an HIV outreach and educational efforts, very few data on HIV risk were available, and only a one-year project conducted at the University of Minnesota (Bockting, Coleman, and Rosser, 1993) was available to use as a resource. Through using GIP peer counselors and GIP participants as informants, we learned that different identity groups within the transgender community needed to hear different messages. As exemplified in the video, many cross-dressers engaged in fantasy role-play in which they tended to disassociate from the reality of risk. Transsexual sex workers were paid more by their customers not to use condoms. Transsexuals in transition were not the only persons sharing needles for hormone injections; some cross-dressers and drag queens were also at risk. Using substances, a risk factor for HIV transmission, cut across all transgender population groups. Transgender men, females to males, did not perceive themselves as at risk, even though many reported engaging in risky sexual practices, such as unprotected oral, vaginal, and anal sex. Transgender persons who were HIV positive needed access to primary care and education about secondary prevention.

PREVENTION STRATEGIES

Several strategies were employed as outreach and education. Through a grant from the New York State AIDS Institute, GIP created a multicultural, multi-identity outreach and education team of peer counselors, who then developed palm cards targeted to transgender women in the sex industry, on the street, and in the club scenes. The image depicted a "fab but not fierce sister" advocating community affiliation and self-care. Peer educators put together safer-sex kits that were packaged in a reusable, clear vinyl cosmetic bag (with different colored trim so it became fashionable to collect one in each color), containing a variety of latex barrier protection, flavored lubes, and a condom guide. The guide is illustrated with "phallic women" demonstrating correct use. Kits also contained lip gloss donated by The Body Shop. Club outreach, house ball outreach, drag event outreach, street outreach, and transgender conference outreach were, and still are, points of dissemination.

The forty-minute video funded by the New York State AIDS Institute focuses on HIV prevention in the context of community building. The making of the video became a community-based education event. Development of the script, hiring of the production crew, locations, interviewees, even the makeup were all tasks of the GIP peer outreach team and other transgender program participants. The video is used as both an educational and training tool, and over 150 copies have been distributed around the world.

Although many of these strategies are still in effect, efforts must constantly be modified to meet emerging needs and respond to lessons learned. Although the safer-sex kits are still quite popular, what is in them has changed. Sex workers need more unlubricated, unflavored condoms for oral sex, and inclusion of chewing gum (with the GIP phone number printed on the package) for after oral sex is greatly appreciated. Dental dams and gloves have been eliminated, since no one reports using them. Outreach workers find that the more they frequent a particular spot, the more likely on the fifth, or sixth, encounter they will have a meaningful conversation and make a successful referral. More concrete services are needed, such as assistance in accessing primary care, benefits, food, and housing. Relationship issues are of great concern—particularly lover and partner issues; and substance use counseling is also needed, with more emphasis on harm reduction and recovery readiness approaches, rather than an abstinence model.

Currently, the Gender Identity Project serves about 1,000 participants annually. Clients tripled since 1995, with GIP participants requesting assistance for many concerns—with housing, benefits, medical and social issues, job-seeking skills, legal issues, and more in-depth counseling for substance use issues, relationship issues, and family concerns. All services include education about HIV, risk reduction and harm reduction counseling, and free condoms and other latex barriers.

TRAINING, ADVOCACY, AND EMPOWERMENT

There continues to be a lack of transgender-sensitive and -relevant treatment services for the whole range of concerns this community faces, especially outpatient and residential substance abuse services. Annually, the GIP conducts an average of fifty sensitivity trainings for social services organizations seeking to better serve transgender clients. Although sensitivity training is a step in the right direction, transgender clients need ongoing services—advocacy, counseling support, and peer groups that the GIP would be better able to offer if more funding for transgender services was available.

To accomplish this, the Lesbian and Gay Community Services Center sees its role in serving the transgender community as more than services delivery. The Gender Identity Project is an opportunity to build leadership in the community that enables transgender activists to speak out on issues of concern, including HIV prevention and intervention, and to take steps toward change. Through the center, GIP Director Rosalyne Blumenstein and GIP peer counselors have also been afforded visibility and a platform from which to advocate to public and private funding sources about the need for developing better resources; to agencies and other organizations about policy changes that will include affirmative services for transgender consumers; and in the community itself, to raise consciousness and activate others. These kinds of activities clearly go beyond the traditional approach, which focuses on changing individual behavior. Facilitating community empowerment to change environments that are oppressive to transgender persons and to establish community norms that advocate HIV prevention should also be the goals of any program or agency serving transgender clients.

REFERENCES

Bockting, W., Coleman, E., and Rosser, S. (1993). *Transgender HIV/AIDS Prevention Program Manual.* Minneapolis: Program in Human Sexuality, Department of Family Practice and Community Health, Medical School, University of Minnesota.

Clements, K., Kitano, K., and Marx, R. (1998). *HIV Prevention and Health Service Needs of the Transgender Community in San Francisco.* Report to the San Francisco Department of Public Health, AIDS Office San Francisco: Department of Public Health.

Elifson, K., Boles, J., Posey, E., Sweat, M., Darrow, W., and Elsea, W. (1993). Male transvestite prostitutes and HIV risk. *American Journal of Public Health* 83(2):260-262.

Mason, T.H., Connors, M., and Kammerer, N. (1995). *Transgender and HIV Risks: Needs Assesment.* Boston: Massachusetts Department of Public Health, AIDS/HIV Bureau.

McKirnan, D.J. and Peterson, P.L. (1989). Alcohol and drug use among homosexual men and women: Epidemiology and population characteristics. *Addictive Behavior* 14(5):545-553.

Positive Health Project (1998). Panel presentation on needle exchange and HIV prevention, AIDS Institute Conference, Albany, NY.

Valentine, D. (1998). *Gender Identity Project Report on Intake Statistics.* New York: Lesbian and Gay Community Services Center of New York and New York University, Department of Anthropology.

Yates, R. (1998). *Male to female sex workers associated risk factors and specific HIV risks, in Group HIV Education for Male To Female Sex Workers: A Facilitators Manual.* Boston: Beacon Hill Multicultural Psychological Associates.

Chapter 10

Sex Reassignment Surgery in HIV-Positive Transsexuals

A. Neal Wilson

INTRODUCTION

The decision to operate on HIV-positive patients was not made by me or my urological colleague; it was made by the ethics committees of the two Detroit Medical Center Hospitals in which we undertake these surgeries. The first case in 1988 turned up with positive serology the day of surgery. Surgery was canceled. The Western blot was positive three days later. The case was presented to the Ethics Committee at the Harper Hospital in the Detroit Medical Center, and this august body deemed it unethical to withhold surgery.

Since that time, eleven HIV-positive transsexual or transgendered individuals have presented to me with a request for sex reassignment surgery. Of these eleven, ten were reassigned. The patient who was not reassigned presented at the age of thirty-seven years, having been in and out of local gender programs for ten years or so, requesting reassignment to "get out of the gay lifestyle." This patient never seriously tried to fulfill the requirements of the Harry Benjamin standards of care. She was diagnosed as HIV positive two years after she first presented to this author. She had many ups and downs and was eventually treated with protease inhibitors. She died of AIDS-related encephalopathy at the age of forty-two. The other ten patients are much more typical.

Correspondence and requests for materials may be sent to A. Neal Wilson, MD, 3011 W. Grand Blvd., Suite 571-5, Detroit, MI 48202.

REVIEW OF LITERATURE

A computerized Medline search of publications from 1966 through the present was conducted and turned up only ten papers concerning HIV positivity and surgery, none of them related to transgendered or transsexual individuals. In 1997, Flum and Wallack[1] conducted a literature search concerning the impact of the human immunodeficiency virus (HIV) infection and syndrome on the practice of surgery. They concluded that the incidence of HIV infection ranges from 1.3 percent of patients hospitalized at sentinel hospitals to 1.5 per 1,000 patients in lower-risk environments. The rate of percutaneous injury during an operation is 5 to 6 percent, and HIV transmission after percutaneous injury with a contaminated needle is .3 percent.

Furthermore, Lowenfels and colleagues[2] reported, in 1993, on the incidence of percutaneous injuries in surgeons. They reported a decrease in the frequency of reported percutaneous injuries over the period 1988 to 1993. The number of yearly injuries per surgeon decreased from 5.5 to 2.1. As Flum and Wallack[1] reported, the transmission of human immunodeficiency virus after percutaneous injury with a needle contaminated with HIV is .3 percent. It would therefore seem not particularly dangerous to the individual surgeon, providing universal precautions are followed, to undertake surgery on HIV-positive patients.

From the first case in 1988 until mid-1995, our index of severity of HIV infection was the CD4 lymphocyte count. After this time, the viral load has been used and this is measured as viral RNA. Before 1995, measurement of viral load was unavailable to us. Currently, I think patients without any history of opportunistic infection, without frank AIDS, with a CD4 lymphocyte count above 200, and with viral replicas less than 600 meet what seems to be the most reasonable parameters for surgery. All these patients present themselves to me thoroughly evaluated by their own doctors, either at home or locally. If they have not been evaluated and no doctor is taking responsibility for their HIV status, then suitable specialists are found for them, either as outpatients or as inpatients certainly, at least during their reassignment surgery. Consultation is undertaken with the patient's primary care doctor, either by telephone or, hopefully, by means of written reports.

FINDINGS

The salient features of the series of eleven are as follows (see also Table 10.1). The age at presentation seeking reassignment surgery varied from nineteen to forty-five years of age with a median age in the late twenties. Of these eleven, most waited one to two years after presentation before reassignment surgery. The number of years of history of HIV-positive status at presentation varied from zero (the patient who turned up positive the morning of surgery, which was then postponed) to nine years, with a median of three years.

The first patient's surgery, when eventually she was rescheduled and the operation was undertaken, was a "Wilson" type procedure involving a corpora cavernosa neurovascular island glans flap, and a skin graft later (see Table 10.2). This was very difficult in this patient, and she sustained a blood loss of 4,500 cc, necessitating fifteen units of packed red cells. Postoperatively she suffered from myglobinemia, renal insufficiency, and femoral neuropathy. This was probably due to the type of operative position in which she was placed. However, she eventually recovered from this and has lived well for the past ten years. Her CD4 count at the time of surgery was 584. No viral load was done on this patient.

Of the remaining nine patients, the operation performed in the succeeding three was a simple penile inversion, on the grounds that this would provide less blood loss and therefore less exposure of the operating room team to the virus. Blood loss for these three averaged just over 700 cc per operation. Blood loss for the more complex Wilson procedure, without including the 4,500 cc loss, averaged 800 to 850 cc. Most hospitalizations were within the expected course, that is, eight to ten days for the penile inversions and fifteen to eighteen days for the Wilson procedures. The renal insufficiency patient was kept in several days longer than the eighteen days. All patients were placed in an intensive care unit (ICU) postoperatively to carefully monitor fluid shifts and blood loss, which in these cases tends to be unpredictable and often severe. The last patient in the series spent six days in the ICU with persistent ooze and required recurrent blood transfusions. There were four late complications in the complete series. One was to repair the labia majora, which had split. The other three suffered from urethral stenosis, which responded to dilatation and foley catherization. The rectum was injured in two cases but healed uneventfully (all patients had a complete bowel prep preop and "triple therapy" antibiotic postoperatively).

TABLE 10.1. Patient Demographics and Summary

Patient initials	0 CR	1 EC	2 WC	3 CS	4 CP	5 TG	6 JT	7 DG	8 LH	9 GS	10 PR
Age at presentation	37	19	25	31	30	34	38	23	29	31	45
Age at SRS	NA	24	27	32	30	35	39	24	31	33	45
Years HIV + at SRS	NA	0	2	7	1	2	1	3	9	7	5
Follow-up (years)	5	10	8	6	6	4	3	3	2	2	0
Comorbid conditions											
IVDA	N	N	N	N	N	N	N	N	N	N	N
Hepatitis B	N	Y	N	N	N	N	Y	Y	N	N	N
Hepatitis C	O	N	N	N	N	N	Y	N	N	N	N
Mortality	42	A&W	A&W	A&W	A&W	39	A&W	A&W	A&W	A&W	A&W

NA   = not applicable
Y   = yes
N   = no
A&W   = alive and well
O   = not available
IVDA = intravenous drug abuser
SRS   = sex reassignment surgery

TABLE 10.2. Hospital Course

Patient initials	SRS Tech.	CD4	Viral Load	Operative Complications	Hospital Course			Late Complications
					T-Max	WBC-Max	Complications	
EC	W	584	NA	Renal insufficiency Myoglobinemia Femeral neuropathy Rectal injury	101	16.9	Renal insufficiency	Partoid hypertrophy
WC	P	51	NA	None	102	WNL	None	Urethral stenosis
CS	P	690	NA	None	101	WNL	Diarrhea (not *Clostridium difficile*)	
CP	P	500	NA	None	WNL	22.9	None	Urethral stenosis
TG	W	156	NA	None	101	WNL	Night sweats	
JT	W	424	NA	None	101	22.2	Chills None	
DG	W	1827	NA	None	102	18.8	Night sweats	Dehiscene of labia majora
LH	W	192	NA	None	102	10.3	None	
GS	W	NA	ND	None	WNL	WNL	None	
PR	W	NA	ND	Rectal injury	101	18.8	None	Urethral stenosis Drug allergy

W   = Wilson technique
P   = penile inversion
WNL = within normal limits
ND = not detectable
NA = not applicable

157

CD4 lymphocyte counts at the time of surgery ranged from 50 all the way up to 1,827, with a median in the 400 to 450 range. One patient with a preoperative CD4 of 304 that decreased to 156 three days postoperatively was treated with intravenous AZT, particularly as she complained of night sweats and chills. This is the only case in the reassigned group of patients who has since died, after having lived four years postsurgery.

Follow-up, either in person or by telephone, indicated that all the patients except the one are alive and well from ten years and one year after their surgery.

Most hospital courses were normal except the renal insufficiency patient and one patient who complained of diarrhea, which was negative for *Clostridium difficile*. The maximum postoperative temperature of the whole series was no more than 102 degrees Fahrenheit. The maximum white blood cell counts for the hospital admissions varied from normal up to 23,000 per cubic centimeter.

In the last two patients, CD4 lymphocyte counts were undertaken but not relied on. Each patient had an undetectable viral load. The three penile inversions were undertaken, as noted previously, on the grounds that less blood loss would expose the operative team to less risk of infection. However, it was pointed out to the author that the Americans with Disabilities Act said, in effect, that there was to be no difference in treatment between HIV-positive patients and normal patients. Therefore, subsequently, we have always undertaken Wilson procedures.[3] Normally, the major reassignment is undertaken on one day; the raw area of the vaginal vault is split skin grafted seven days later; the skin graft is then looked at seven days after this (fifteen days postop); and the patient is sent home within the next few days if everything is fine. It is possible to split skin graft the vaginal vault at the same time as the original procedure, thus possibly shortening the hospitalization to eight to ten days, but the reliability of the skin graft take is much less. The author has received one or two requests so far for a rectosigmoid neocalphorrhapy in the HIV-positive patient. After lengthy discussion with the general surgeons who undertake this surgery and the ethics committees, it was decided that this would not be justifiable at this time.

CONCLUSION

It seems there are no predictors concerning the patients who will do poorly after surgery. Night sweats are a fairly commonly described symptom and these were mentioned by four or five of our patients. It should be noted, however, that only the one who died described this in detail as "running rivers of ice over my back." The patient who's CD4 lymphocyte count was only fifty-one at operation subsequently went on to an almost zero CD4 lymphocyte count. This was managed with protease inhibitors, and the patient, on last speaking with her on the telephone, asserted that she was alive and doing well and her CD4 lymphocyte count was in the 350 range. In conclusion, provided certain criteria are met, HIV-positive transsexuals can undergo sex reassignment surgery.

NOTES

1. Flum, D.R., and Wallack, M.K. (1997). The surgeon's database for AIDS: A collective review. *Journal of the American College of Surgeons* 184(4):403-412.

2. Lowenfels, A.B., Mehta,V., Levi,.D.A., Montecalvo, M.A., Savino, J.A., and Wormer, G.P. (1933). Reduced frequency of percutaneous injuries in surgeons. *AIDS* 9(2):199-202.

3. The details of the Wilson procedure have been available on the Internet for some time. The procedure itself has not been published in hard-form copy as it is still evolving. Basically, the perineum is opened with the posterior perineal skin flap and the vagina is constructed. Bilateral orchiectomies are undertaken; the scrotum and penile skin are split in the midline, leaving a rectangular penile skin flap; the penis itself is dissected leaving the urethra and spongiosis ventral and separate; one-third of one corpus cavernosa is dissected out and left to carry the vascular supply and nerve supply to a small segment of the original glans. The reconstruction is begun by first suturing in the posterior perineal skin flap; then suturing in the penile skin flap to the prostatic fascia and at each side to the posterior perineal skin flap; then bringing through the urethra and the glans of the clitoris, bringing down the labia scrotal elements, and suturing them to the midline. The raw vaginal vault is skin grafted one week later. A first graft dressing change is undertaken one week after this. The main advantage is that there is enough penile skin left on the outside to undertake reconstruction of the labia minora and clitoral hood. The bulb of the penis can be removed later, and the urinary stream adjusted to suit the patient. The clitoral shaft and the glans apparatus comes from above downward rather than below upward, as in the simple penile inversions with the residual urethra. Erotic sensation to the glans is preserved.

Chapter 11

Guidelines for Selecting
HIV-Positive Patients
for Genital Reconstructive Surgery

Sheila Kirk

INTRODUCTION

Surgery is often thought of in two distinctly different contexts—
surgical procedures that are indicated and surgery that is designated
as elective. Indicated surgery inherently carries the concept of a need,
based on emergency or urgency, and is an approach to a cure or that
which has the capacity to restore to health, or as close to it as possible.
Elective procedures in surgery, particularly in some specialties, have
not so vigorous a need and may even have a need that can be delayed
or put off indefinitely. Urgency is not something associated with the
word "elective."

When we apply the words "indicated" and "elective" to the transgender community, particularly the transsexual person, we could
draw argument from a number of people. Transsexuals, both male-to-female
and female-to-male will refuse to accept the term elective. For them,
it is never elective but always indicated. And in many respects, they
are correct. Genital reconstructive surgery (GRS) to accomplish con-
gruity between mind, spirit, and body, between identity and anatomy
is truly indicated in my view as well, but not so in the opinion of many
professionals. Many caretakers think of it as an option and not a necessity. This concept is quite different from the opinions of sur-
gery-seeking transsexuals. Fixing one's nose or jaw, reshaping the

torso or the hairline could much more probably be considered elective in most individuals' thinking, including my own. I raise these points in consideration of the transsexual because a percentage of transsexual individuals are in a conditon of ill health that is particularly grave. I refer to the transsexual who is a very apt candidate for genital reconstructive surgery from a psychologic standpoint but who is HIV-positive. While I believe them to have a place in the indicated surgical patient group and to not belong to an elective surgical group, they do have an important underlying health concern that needs to be examined closely, with not only great consideration and planning but with the cooperative effort and expertise of a number of professionals.

There is very little in the surgical literature about transgendered persons who are HIV-positive undergoing genital reassignment. One has to read surgical reports of nontransgendered HIV-positive individuals having surgery that is usually performed for emergency or urgency reasons. Hence, guidelines for preoperative assessment of the HIV-positive transgender person are not discussed in the literature to any extent. It is very important to establish some criteria, even at the risk of my being somewhat academic. It is important to establish a preoperative protocol because of two deeply concerning ideas, of which I am aware, that are somewhat evident in some surgeons' views.

First, the opinion of many is that HIV-positive patients are to be considered just the same as anyone else; hence, special precautions with selection of procedure, allowing heavy acute blood loss, and management of intraoperative and postoperative infection are no more a consideration than for anyone else. In my view, that can be a dangerous idea. HIV-positive patients deserve to be treated as normal, that is true. But they cannot be altogether because of the nature of the virus they carry and its potential for serious consequences.

The second practice many surgeons follow involves discontinuance of antiretroviral therapy before surgery and the casual and often delayed return to the therapeutic regimen that was in use before the procedure. This is an observed practice of some surgeons who performed surgery of various kinds for HIV-positive individuals. It came to my attention while serving in a large HIV medical practice. The nature of the medical regimen is often ignored, with no realization that some antiretrovirals cannot be discontinued for more than a day or two for fear of viral strain resistance (i.e., Crixivan [indinavir sulfate][1,2]).

Basic ignorance in these two areas leads one to believe that other nuances and refinements in readying a patient for a three- to four-hour procedure, such as a vaginoplasty for a male-to-female individual, are not known. In addition, although postreassignment convalescence often can be most uncomplicated, the threat of pulmonary, operative site, and urinary tract infections exists even more so in this population. These individuals, if not stable and well controlled in their HIV status, are very susceptible and can develop serious postoperative complications.

With these thoughts in mind, it is important to consider some guidelines that should be part of the preoperative evaluation of the HIV-infected transsexual. The gathering of information about an HIV-infected patient can be somewhat involved, but it harkens back to a very important surgical concept that must never be forgotten. Preoperative selection and preparation strongly influences surgical outcome. When we are dealing with patients who have excellent reasons for having their surgery but do not have to rush into it until they are properly assessed and prepared, the concept becomes even more cogent.

GUIDELINES

1. Contact with primary physician caring for patient's HIV disease
2. Evaluation of medical history of the disease in the patient
3. Evaluation of lab data from the past, and a discussion of the most recent treatment regimen and the patient's response

Contact with the Primary Physician

Identifying the medical physician who cares for the HIV patient seeking genital reconstruction is most important. In-depth conversation with this professional is vital. That doctor can trace the history of this patient's infection, giving important information about opportunistic illness, infections, other sexually transmitted diseases, and sarcoma as well as treatment plans that have failed and been replaced and those which have been effective. He or she can give important information about recent laboratory data and, in the process of information exchange, give insight into the patient's reliability to keep appointments and to follow instructions in treatment regimens and, most important, into behavioral changes that can lead to good health practices. A striking phenomenon develops sometimes when patients exercise denial of their disorder and stop treatment or when their use of alcohol and other organ-damaging substances continues and/or worsens. It is particularly upsetting to observe patients take a new lover who is also HIV-positive and then abandon not only safe-sex practices but even the antiretroviral regimens that have been so effective, believing nothing more can take place to worsen this or any other disease process. Patients can develop new strains of virus resistant to the previously successful regimen just by cohabiting with someone infected with different strains, especially when neither uses safe-sex practices.[3] This health care provider is essential in the circle of care to be established before a surgical date is determined. That initial conversation others will lead to others, and requests should be made for transfer of records, at least for the past year and, if possible, for previous years if need be.

Evaluation of Transferred Medical History

Upon receipt of medical records, which should include both office and relevant hospital records, the task of evaluation can become difficult, yet it must be thorough. Pertinent information must include the following:

- The time interval since diagnosis was first made to the present, with pertinent medical/surgical events detailed
- The kinds of infection experienced in that time, and, in particular, modes of treatment along with levels of response and success in treatment
- Details of hospitalizations with diagnosis of illnesses, treatment, and response
- Antiretroviral regimens in the past, and their success or failure, as indicated by the patient's health status and lab data in those time periods
- Details of current antiretroviral regimen: how long in place, viral loads, and CD4 counts with this particular regimen
- A review of CD4 counts and viral load counts for the past six months to a year
- Details about other systems' involvement, i.e., central nervous system, liver function, as well as eye or pulmonary dysfunction or infections[4]

- Other medications being used and their effectiveness; whether antibiotic prophylaxis, psychotropic medication, androgens, Marinol, etc., are being used
- The daily activity level of this patient; whether the patient is employed or not, in therapy, or engaged in volunteer work

Evaluation of Lab Data, Most Recent Treatment Regimen, and the Patient's Response

Looking at liver and kidney function testing for the past year and to the present time is very helpful. Subtle trends can be seen, and any patient demonstrating even gradual failure in these systems may not be a candidate for genital reconstructive surgery. Special liver and kidney studies may be indicated, including needle biopsy, and if there is a history of alcohol abuse and/or hepatitis, these studies are mandatory.

A detailed evaluation of CD4/CD8 cells is most important as an indicator of T cell resilience and capacity to return to acceptable levels. Has the patient had inability to maintain red blood cell counts and proper indices in different regimens? What has been the response to treatment? What is the current viral load? Is there a positive trend? Is it in the undetectable range, that is below 400 copies? And with refined viral measurement technique, what is the actual count below 400? Have viral loads been effectively lowered with a change in antiretroviral medication in the past, and if so, for how long?[4,5] What antiretrovirals have been used in the natural history of the infection in a particular patient, and with what success for the patient's quality of health and longevity of life? One may need a full year of laboratory studies to formulate a pattern for patient stability.

MY PERSONAL EXPERIENCE

The author is a surgeon who, for a considerable time, performed and assisted in a surgical practice where over 130 genital reassignment patients were operated upon, among them five HIV-positive male-to-female transsexuals. In addition to genital reassignment, one of the group underwent breast augmentation as well. None had facial cosmetic surgery. The series is small, without doubt, but experience with them has served strongly to formulate our evaluative policy for this very deserving portion of our transgender patient caseload. We have followed the guidelines outlined to the letter, and this very carefully observed policy has led to completely uncomplicated intraoperative experience and a particularly complication-free postoperative course, both in the acute as well as the intermediate postoperative period. None of our patients have received blood or developed infection. Our plan, though detailed, is a simple one. It means being meticulous and willing to exchange with the health care provider who is actively managing the patient applying to us. Our goal was to determine that these patients experienced stability, good health, and acceptable laboratory values before surgery for a significant period of time. Their CD4 cells had to be at least 200 cells per millimeter, and preferably 300 or more. Viral loads had to be 400 copies per milliliter or below, and these studies had to be at these levels for at least three months on the current antiretroviral regimen. These patients demonstrated excellent liver and kidney function for at least a year, and in that year, opportunistic disease did not occur or, if it did, was perhaps no more than mild herpes simplex or zoster outbreaks. Our first patient is now about nine months postoperative, very well and very stable in her disease. The others report good stable health patterns, although more time will be necessary for adequate follow-up.

One of our very important approaches was to reinstitute the preoperative antiretroviral regimen as quickly as possible after surgery. The last preoperative dosage is given about four hours before the usual morning administration time, and well before the surgical start time. The next dosage is given with no more delay than six hours after the usual midday or late-day dose. Regimens in general involve a three-drug therapy, requiring specific times of day for taking the drugs. Some drugs are once-a-day regimens, facilitating the continuance of the therapy. On the day of surgery, after the procedure, the "at-home" medical physician responsible for HIV care is called and given a report. Another report is made to that doctor within forty-eight hours. There is a highly skilled team of HIV specialists in the city of Pittsburgh, with whom the author of this paper practiced for two years. They were available for consultation, though it was never needed.

We ask our patients to bring their own medication, the entire daily regimen and, most important, the antiviral medications. Once they are judged able to begin taking their own medications, we entrust them to reinstitute the program of self-medication as determined by their "at-home" medical doctor. Our nursing staff generally does not administer medications, except for one or two occasions after the operation, although they do keep track to ensure that the patient does not omit any part of the regimen. Allowing our patients to restart self-administration of their medication regimen quickly encourages them to take responsibility for their wellness and well-being.[5]

CONCLUSION

Because a patient is HIV positive, the door need not be closed to a surgical procedure to assist in accomplishing a congruence between body and mind. Even surgeries for facial cosmetic purposes or body contouring are appropriate to consider for such a patient. While it is not my experience in this regard as yet, some surgeons do feel it is important to consider.[6] The word "elective" is not an appropriate one, in our view, when considering the needs of the transgender person for candidacy in our surgical center. What is appropriate is thoroughness in evaluation and assuring that the surgical candidate will not suffer increased harm due to his or her HIV disease if human endeavor can in any way prevent it. Heretofore, surgeons performing surgery for the transsexual eliminated the HIV-positive person from consideration. This should not be so. Granted, not all will be candidates, but thoughtful selection can be applied and can transform some individual's crushed dreams to quality living and fulfillment.

At the Harry Benjamin International Gender Dysphoria Association's convention held in Vancouver in September 1997, members endorsed a policy that favored surgery for the HIV-infected transsexual. No guidelines were formulated then, nor have any been since. Our hope is that the precepts outlined in this paper will fortify that policy and help GRS surgeons consider this special population for the treatment and care they deserve.

NOTES

1. Personal Communication, Merck and Company Pharmaceuticals, Research Division Director, June 1998.

2. Personal Communication, DuPont Pharmaceuticals, Research Director, July 1998.

3. Condra, J.H., Schleif, W.A., Blahy, O.M., Gabryelski, L.J., Graham, D.J., Quintero, J.C., Rhodes, A., Robbins, H.L., Roth, E., and Shivaprakash, M. et al.

(1995). In vivo emergence of HIV-1 variants resistant to multiple protease inhibitors. *Nature* 374(6522):569-571.

4. Mellors, J.W., Munoz, A., Giorgi, J.V., Margolick, J.B., Tassoni, C.J., Gupta, P., Kingsley, L.A., Todd, J.A., Saah, A.J., Detels, R., Phair, J.P., and Rinaldo, C.R., Jr. (1997). Plasma viral load and CD4 lymphocytes as prognostic markers of HIV-1 infection. *Annals of Internal Medicine.* 126(12):946-954.

5. O'Brien, W.A., Hartigan, P.M., Martin, D., Esinhart, J., Hill, A., Benoit, S., Rubin, M., Simberkoff, M.S., and Hamilton, J.D. (1996). Changes in plasma HIV-1 RNA and CD4 lymphocyte counts and the risk of progression to AIDS. *New England Journal of Medicine.* 334(25):426-431.

6. Hage, J.J., Vossen, M., and Becking, A.G. (1997). Rhinoplasty, a part of gender confirming surgery in male transsexuals: Basic considerations and clinical experience. *Annals of Plastic Surgery.* 39(3)(September):266-271.

Index

Page numbers followed by the letter "n" indicate notes; those followed by the letter "t" indicate tables.

Prevention materials, 83-84
Prevention strategies, 14-15, 30-32,
    51-52, 108-109
Prevention workshops, 104-111
Prieur, A., 115n5, 116n21
Prince, V., 12n7
Prison, 43-44, 75, 85
Prostitutes, 45, 53. *See also* Sex work
Prostitution, 2, 19-20, 27-28, 33-34n8,
    49, 75-76. *See also* Sex work
PROVIVA [Project Informing You
    About the AIDS Virus], 3
Proyecto ContraSIDA Por Vida, 69
Psychological issues, of transgenders,
    26, 44, 116n16
Pugh, K., 66
PWAC of New York, 46

Quadland, M., 133
Qualitative evaluation, 135
Quantitative evaluation, 134-135
Queen, use of term, 33n5
"Queen of Denial," 26
Queer, expansion of term, 41
Quinn, T.C., 34n10
Quintero, J.C., 167n3

Ramos, R., 123
Ray, S., 34n11
Raymond, J., 16, 18, 45
Reback, C.J., *xxi,* 59, 65, 66
Reciprocal collaboration, 139
Recruitment of transgenders for
    workshop, 126-127
Reeza, G., 98n1
Rejection, transgenders' fears of, 42
Rekart, M.L., 66
Remafedi, G., 26
Researchers, collaboration with
    community, 122-123, 140
Reter, D.J., 138
Rezza, G., 12n9
Rhodes, A., 167n3
Rhodes, F., 24
Rice, M., 99n15
Richards, Jennifer, 137

Rickert, V.I., 124
Rietmeijer, C.A., 122, 124
Rinaldo, C.R., Jr., 167n4
Rio de Janeiro, culture of *travestismo*
    in, 1-12
Risk, conceptualization of, 21-25
Risk Behavior Assessment (RBA)
    interview instrument, 5, 9
Risk Behavior Follow-Up Assessment
    (RBFA) interview instrument, 5
Risk category, 21
Risk factors for HIV
    of male transvestite sex workers in
        Brazil, 7-8, 8t
    marginalization, 14
    psychological factors, 26
    silicone injections, 9-10
    social and cultural, 105-106
Risk group, 14, 21
Risk management, 108-109, 110-111
Risk reduction, 108-109
Risk structures, 22-23, 25-29
Robbins, H.L., 167n3
Robinson, B.E., *xix, xx,* 26, 98n1, 120,
    125, 134, 136
Robinson, E., 89n4
Rofes, E., 116n13
Romyen, S., 34n8
Rosenstock, I.M., 128
Rosie's Place, 43
Rosser, B.R.S.
    on affirmation of gender identity,
        128
    on clients of transgendered sex
        workers, 24
    on evaluation of prevention
        program, 134, 136
    on identity affirmation, 29
    on lack of prevention programs,
        xix
    on needs assessment, 125
    on participant satisfaction with
        workshop, 135
    on prevention program in
        Minnesota, *xxii,* 46, 119, 148
    on prevention workers' lack of
        knowledge, *xx*

Treatment regimen, evaluating before
    surgery, 165
Treichler, P.A., 22
Tri-Ess, 138
Trust, between participants and
    facilitator, 106, 138-139
Tucker, P., 66
Tulvatana, S., 34n8
Twelve-step programs, 32, 43

University of Minnesota Program in
    Human Sexuality, *xix, xx*
Unprotected sex, 76-78
Unsterilized needles, and hormone
    injections, 20-21
U.S. Centers for Disease Control and
    Prevention, 59

Valdiserri, R.O., 122, 139
Valentine, D., 41, 147
Valenzi, C., 12n9, 98n1
Van Maasdam, J., 138
Van Ness Prevention Division (VNPD),
    60
Van Ness Recovery House Prevention
    Division, 59
Vectors, as epidemiological concept, 25
Videos
    affirming transgender expression
        and promoting condom use, 134
    documentary of transsexual men,
        102
    eroticizing safer sex, 133
    HIV prevention, 145
    personalizing HIV/AIDS, 131-132
VNPD Transgender Harm Reduction
    Program, 60-61
    participants' alcohol and drug use,
        62, 63t
    participants' demographics, 62, 63t
    participants' injection drug use
        and risks, 64t
    sex work of participants, 64-66
Vonsover, A., 66

Vossen, M., 167n6
Vulva Riot, 138

Walker, C.M., 122, 123
Wallack, M.K., 154
Ward, T.P., 24
Warren, B.E., *xxiii*, 145
Wawer, M.J., 25
Weeks, J., 22
Welfare, 44
West Hollywood (CA), prevention
    program in, 59-68
Wilchins, Riki Ann, 145
Wilkinson, W., *xxii*
Willms, D., 122, 139
Wilson, A.N., *xxiii*, 153
Wilson procedure, 155, 157t, 158, 159n3
Wingood, G.M., 123, 124
Withers, K., 31, 46
Wodak, A., 99n16
*Women, Poverty, and AIDS: Sex,
    Drugs, and Structural Violence*
    (Farmer, Connors, and
    Simmons), 30
Wong, M.L., 121
Wood, M.M., 24
Woodhouse, A., 18, 34n13, 40
Work. *See* Employment
Workshop curriculum, 129t
Workshops, 127
Wormer, G.P., 154
Wright, N., 34n8

Yates, R., 146
Yep, G.A., 89n8
*You Don't Know Dick: Courageous
    Hearts of Transsexual Men*, 102
Youth Enrichment Services (YES), 147

Zaccarelli, M., 12n9, 98n1
Zevin, B., 89n3
Zigler, E., 26
Zinn, M., 66

Order Your Own Copy of
This Important Book for Your Personal Library!

TRANSGENDER AND HIV
Risks, Prevention, and Care

_____in hardbound at $49.95 (ISBN: 0-7890-1267-7)

_____in softbound at $24.95 (ISBN: 0-7890-1268-5)

COST OF BOOKS_____

OUTSIDE USA/CANADA/
MEXICO: ADD 20%____

POSTAGE & HANDLING_____
(US: $4.00 for first book & $1.50
for each additional book)
Outside US: $5.00 for first book
& $2.00 for each additional book)

SUBTOTAL_____

in Canada: add 7% GST____

STATE TAX____
(NY, OH & MIN residents, please
add appropriate local sales tax)

FINAL TOTAL____
(If paying in Canadian funds,
convert using the current
exchange rate, UNESCO
coupons welcome.)

❏ **BILL ME LATER:** ($5 service charge will be added)
(Bill-me option is good on US/Canada/Mexico orders only;
not good to jobbers, wholesalers, or subscription agencies.)

❏ Check here if billing address is different from
shipping address and attach purchase order and
billing address information.

Signature_____

❏ **PAYMENT ENCLOSED: $**_____

❏ **PLEASE CHARGE TO MY CREDIT CARD.**

❏ Visa   ❏ MasterCard   ❏ AmEx   ❏ Discover
❏ Diner's Club   ❏ Eurocard   ❏ JCB

Account # _____

Exp. Date_____

Signature_____

Prices in US dollars and subject to change without notice.

NAME_____

INSTITUTION_____

ADDRESS_____

CITY_____

STATE/ZIP_____

COUNTRY_____ COUNTY (NY residents only)_____

TEL_____ FAX_____

E-MAIL_____

May we use your e-mail address for confirmations and other types of information? ❏ Yes ❏ No
We appreciate receiving your e-mail address and fax number. Haworth would like to e-mail or fax special
discount offers to you, as a preferred customer. **We will never share, rent, or exchange your e-mail address
or fax number.** We regard such actions as an invasion of your privacy.

Order From Your Local Bookstore or Directly From
The Haworth Press, Inc.
10 Alice Street, Binghamton, New York 13904-1580 • USA
TELEPHONE: 1-800-HAWORTH (1-800-429-6784) / Outside US/Canada: (607) 722-5857
FAX: 1-800-895-0582 / Outside US/Canada: (607) 722-6362
E-mail: getinfo@haworthpressinc.com
PLEASE PHOTOCOPY THIS FORM FOR YOUR PERSONAL USE.
www.HaworthPress.com

BOF00